EYE AND VISION RESEARCH DEVELOPMENTS

CONJUNCTIVITIS

ETIOLOGY, DIAGNOSIS AND CLINICAL MANAGEMENT

EYE AND VISION RESEARCH DEVELOPMENTS

Additional books in this series can be found on Nova's website under the Series tab.

Additional e-books in this series can be found on Nova's website under the e-book tab.

EYE AND VISION RESEARCH DEVELOPMENTS

CONJUNCTIVITIS

ETIOLOGY, DIAGNOSIS AND CLINICAL MANAGEMENT

ELIAS H. BAZILE
EDITOR

NOVA BIOMEDICAL
New York

For permission to use material from this book please contact us:
Telephone 631-231-7269; Fax 631-231-8175
Web Site: http://www.novapublishers.com

Library of Congress Cataloging-in-Publication Data

Library of Congress Control Number: 2014946015

ISBN: 978-1-63321-621-1

Published by Nova Science Publishers, Inc. † New York

CONTENTS

PREFACE

Conjunctivitis is a common ocular problem that can be seen worldwide and it is still under consideration for global public health. There are many causes of conjunctivitis. Clinically, bacterial conjunctivitis is characterized by purulent ocular discharge, eye crusting or sticky eyes on awakening, foreign body sensation, and conjunctival injection. In more severe cases, chemosis and lid edema may also occur. The involvement is usually unilateral at first but rapidly spreads to the contralateral eye. There are also many tropical infections and disorders that can induce conjunctivitis and those problems are called tropical conjunctivitis. This book discusses several causes of different cases of conjunctivitis. It provides information on the etiology, the diagnosis of different forms of conjunctivitis, and the clinical management.

Chapter 1 – Properly speaking, blepharitis is the inflammation of the lid margin. Although the term is often applied loosely according to etymology (βλέφαρον, eyelid) to pathologic phenomena interesting the whole eyelid, this should called eyelid dermatitis; "blepharitis" is best reserved to describe the alteration of the border zone between skin and conjunctiva. This is the meeting point of two highly correlated, reciprocally influencing biological domains. Blepharitis can be acute or chronic. Particularly, chronic blepharitis (CB) is a bothering condition with heavy implications on quality of life. It can apparently start from the cutaneous side, with seborrheic or infectious-ulcerative features interesting the eyebrows, and Zeis's and Moll's glands; or from the conjunctival one, with complex, and yet poorly understood dysfunctions of Meibomian glands and of the lachrymal film. CB can subsist by itself, or can be regarded as a resulting stage inscribed in the syndrome of several oculocutaneous diseases, typically rosacea. It can be difficult to distinguish whether CB is a primary process; or, on the contrary, whether is a specific manifestation of an underlying dermatological condition. More important, CB is cause of embarrass to dermatologists, who often are not aware how to deal with it. The author will discuss diagnosis, differerential, as well as treatment, either approved or of the "tips-and-tricks" kind.

Chapter 2 – Infectious crystalline keratopathy (ICK), first described in 1983, is a corneal infection characterized by branching, white, crystalline opacities within the corneal stroma and occasionally with anterior segment inflammation, with or without epithelial defect. Neither racial nor gender predisposition have been described. Risk factors for infectious crystalline keratopathy include long-term topical corticosteroid use, previous corneal surgery, prior corneal disease, systemic immunocompromised disorder and local anesthetic abuse. Diagnosis of ICK is basically established by clinical appearance on slit-lamp examination, but the isolation of microorganisms may improve the effectiveness of treatment. It is not easy to isolate the agent, the infiltrate may often lie deep into the corneal stroma, and deep corneal scrapings or corneal biopsy may be required. Numerous microorganisms have been identified as causative agents, such as gram positive alpha hemolytic aerobic streptococcus (being the most common Streptoccocus viridans), staphylococcus (such as Staphilo-ccocus aureus and Haemolyticus), fungi, pseudomonas, mycobacterium, peptostreptococcus, corynebacterium, proprionobacterium and acanthamoeba. Differential diagnoses of ICK including fungal keratitis, bacterial keratitis, herpes simplex keratitis, graft rejection, Schnyder's dystrophy and multiple myeloma. First step treatment consists in topical antibiotics with bactericidal activity, such as vancomycin or other potent antibiotic agents with good gram-positive coverage, depending on culture or biopsy results. Response to medication is poor and slow because the bacteria are enveloped in a biofilm isolating the infectious organisms from the antimicrobial penetration. Some reports suggest the use of systemic antibiotics in severe cases. In absence of response antifungal therapy should be considered. Penetrating keratoplasty or lamellar keratectomy in patients with corneal scarring involving visual axis due to ICK may be helpful for visual rehabilitation.

Chapter 3 – Objectives: Ambient air pollution exposure has been associated with the occurrence of several different health conditions.

These associations are not only limited to respiratory and cardiovascular system; there have been also number of studies that have linked ambient air pollutions to non-respiratory conditions, such as cardiac disease, appendicitis, headaches and migraines, skin conditions, eye discomfort and conjunctivitis. The purpose of this study was to examine the associations between emergency department (ED) visits for conjunctivitis and ambient air pollution levels in Calgary, Alberta, Canada.

Materials and Methods: The National Ambulatory Care Reporting System was used to obtain patient information on ED visits for conjunctivitis for the period of January 2010 to December 2011. ED visits for conjunctivitis were defined using the International Classification of Diseases, Tenth revision (ICD-10) codes H10. A time stratified case-crossover design was applied in this study. Odds ratios (ORs) and their 95% confidence intervals (95%CI) for emergency department visits were calculated for one unit increase in each pollutant (nitrogen dioxide (NO_2), fine particulate matter with a median aerodynamic diameter of less than 2.5 μm ($PM_{2.5}$) and ozone (O_3)), controlling for temperature and relative humidity.

Results: Among 4,333 ED visits for conjunctivitis (49% females, 51% males), analyses were conducted considering cold weather months (October to March) and warm weather months (April to September). During the warm months, statistically significant positive results were observed in the female population for NO_2 and for lags 5-7 days, with the highest result for lag 5 days (OR = 1.048; 95%CI = 1.020, 1.076) and in the male population for $PM_{2.5}$ lagged 6 days (OR = 1.014; 95%CI = 1.002, 1.026). During the cold months, statistically significant positive results were observed for females and NO_2 lagged 7 days (OR = 1.021; 95%CI = 1.001, 1.040) and for $PM_{2.5}$ for lag 2 days (OR = 1.042; 95%CI = 1.004, 1.079) and for males and O_3 lagged 5 and 6 days, with the highest result for lag 6 (OR = 1.035; 95%CI = 1.009, 1.062).

Conclusion: The findings of this study suggest that there are associations between level of air pollution and ED visits for conjunctivitis in Calgary, Canada. The authors' findings support associations reported in the literature for NO_2 among females. The latency period between exposure and ED visit for conjunctivitis in this study coincides with the typical incubation period for infectious conjunctivitis.

Chapter 4 – Bacterial conjunctivitis is common in childhood and accounts for 1 to 2% of primary care encounters. In the neonatal period, the most common causative organism is *Staphylococcus aureus* followed by *Chlamydia trachomatis*. Other organisms include *Haemophilus influenzae*, *Streptococcus pneumoniae*, and *Neisseria gonorrhoeae*. In children, bacterial conjunctivitis is most often caused by *H. influenzae*, *S. pneumoniae*, and *Moraxella catarrhalis*. Clinically, bacterial conjunctivitis is characterized by purulent ocular discharge, eye crusting or sticky eyes on awakening, foreign body sensation, and conjunctival injection. In more severe cases, chemosis and lid edema may also occur. The involvement is usually unilateral at first but rapidly spreads to the contralateral eye. The diagnosis is mainly clinically. Cultures along with Gram or Giemsa stains should be considered in neonatal conjunctivitis, conjunctivitis presenting with severe purulent discharge, suspected venereal infections, immunodeficiency, recurrent cases, or cases that fail to respond to therapy. While it is beyond doubt that conjunctivitis caused by *C. trachomatis* or *N. gonorrhoeae* needs to be treated, some authors suggest a watchful observation approach to other bacterial causes of conjunctivitis as most other cases of bacterial conjunctivitis are self-limited. A recent Cochrane review, however, suggests that the use of antibiotic eye drops is associated with modestly improved rates of clinical and microbiological remission in comparison to the use of placebo. The present consensus supports prompt use of topical antibiotics as they shorten the course of the disease, reduce the discomfort associated with the infection, reduce the risk of ocular damage, prevent person-to-person transmission, and reduce rate of re-infection.

Chapter 5 – of severely painful conjunctivitis and subconjunctival hemorrhage. Coxsackievirus A24 variant and Enterovirus 70 are the major etiological agents involved in acute hemorrhagic conjunctivitis. The first outbreak of acute hemorrhagic conjunctivitis was described in 1969 in Ghana, West Africa. A second focus appeared in Java (Indonesia) in 1969-70. Since then, both viruses have spread to five continents in a pandemic fashion over 45 years and are now an important world public health problem. This chapter provides a state-of-the-art review of the major aspects of the etiology, diagnosis, and clinical management and control measures of acute hemorrhagic conjunctivitis.

Chapter 6 – Conjunctivitis is a common ocular problem that can be seen worldwide and it is still under consideration for global public health. There are many causes of conjunctivitis. The interesting group of conjunctivitis disorders is those found in tropical zone. There are many tropical infections and disorders that can induce conjunctivitis and those problems are called tropical conjunctivitis. In this short article, the authors will summarize and discuss on important kinds of tropical conjunctivitis focusing on diagnosis and management.

In: Conjunctivitis
Editor: Elias H. Bazile

ISBN: 978-1-63321-621-1

Chapter 1

THE BLEPHARITIS CONUNDRUM: A DERMATOLOGICAL VIEWPOINT ON DIAGNOSIS AND PRACTICAL MANAGEMENT

Giovanni Luigi Capella, MD*
Milan, Italy

ABSTRACT

Properly speaking, blepharitis is the inflammation of the lid margin. Although the term is often applied loosely according to etymology (βλέφαρον, eyelid) to pathologic phenomena interesting the whole eyelid, this should called eyelid dermatitis; "blepharitis" is best reserved to describe the alteration of the border zone between skin and conjunctiva. This is the meeting point of two highly correlated, reciprocally influencing biological domains. Blepharitis can be acute or chronic. Particularly, chronic blepharitis (CB) is a bothering condition with heavy implications on quality of life. It can apparently start from the cutaneous side, with seborrheic or infectious-ulcerative features interesting the eyebrows, and Zeis's and Moll's glands; or from the conjunctival one, with complex, and yet poorly understood dysfunctions of Meibomian

* Author's address: Giovanni Luigi Capella, MD, Private practice, Dermatology & STD, 7, Via Sauli Sant'Alessandro, 20127, Milan, Italy, phone: +39-(0)2-2822542, e-mail: progderm @ katamail.com

glands and of the lachrymal film. CB can subsist by itself, or can be regarded as a resulting stage inscribed in the syndrome of several oculocutaneous diseases, typically rosacea. It can be difficult to distinguish whether CB is a primary process; or, on the contrary, whether is a specific manifestation of an underlying dermatological condition. More important, CB is cause of embarrass to dermatologists, who often are not aware how to deal with it. The author will discuss diagnosis, differerential, as well as treatment, either approved or of the "tips-and-tricks" kind.

INTRODUCTION

Properly speaking, *blepharitis* is the inflammation of the margin of eyelids (Duke-Elder and MacFaul, 1974; Trevor-Roper, 1974; Newell, 1978). Although, according to plain etymology (βλέφαρον, the whole eyelid), the term is often loosely applied to pathologic phenomena interesting or extending to the cutaneous side of the eyelid(s), such processes should be referred to as *eyelid dermatitis* (Parkinson, 1996). Indeed, "blepharitis" is best reserved to describe the inflammatory involvement of the lid border zone between skin and conjunctiva. Somehow cumbersomely, some authors admit the term "blepharitis" to designate whole lid dermatitis, and call "ciliary" or "marginal blepharitis" the inflammation of the lid border (Toselli and Miglior, 1979; Czepita et al., 2007). This is a highly specialized anatomical district with a mucocutaneous junction, akin to other sites such as the mouth, the nose, the anogenital orifices (Bron et al., 2011a), all of which are characterized by similar epithelial transitions between mucosa and the skin. Blepharitides are arbitrarily divided into acute and chronic, anterior and posterior, but such distinctions are not clear-cut and can be misleading: indeed, these disease processes are often chronic but flare-ups can ensue, either from the basic etiology or from superimposed worsening factors, especially environmental ones. Moreover, "real-world" cases, especially advanced ones, refrain from neat topographical stratification. Dermatologists are ill at ease with blepharitis, and are prone to commit all these cases directly to ophthalmologists, thus abdicating their consultant role, and possibly missing some diagnostic, therapeutic, and research opportunities, in spite of the fact that blepharitis, especially the chronic form, is quite frequent in dermatological patients (Auw-Haedrich and Reinhard, 2007). This brief chapter has been written by a clinical dermatologist bored of finding himself "ill at ease" with this ticklish topic, and is humbly intended to fill an educational gap.

1. Acute Blepharitis: Not Always Quite Trivial

Acute blepharitis (AB - "inflammation *of lids* with rapid onset" [Hampton Roy, 1993] – note how the above pointed terminological mistake is perpetuated even in authoritative textbooks) is often a self-explaining process ensuing from evident etiologies mainly involving the surrounding eyelid skin or conjunctiva. "Acute" refers not only to onset celerity, but also to intensity of manifestations. The eye is red rimmed, secretion and lacrimation can be copious, and the patient complains of pruritus or, more often, of burning sensation or even frank pain. AB can be the expression of *allergic* or *irritant contact dermatitis,* flares of *atopic dermatitis*, *herpes simplex* or *zoster*, *phthiriasis*, and virtually any bacterial, fungine, or viral infection (Table 1). Dirt and staphylococci stand out as causes of AB in children: the classical clinical expression in such settings is *follicular impetiginous AB* (Duke-Elder and MacFaul, 1974). New entries include allergic blepharitis due to eyelash extension, which are applied with glues containing formaldehyde (Amano et al., 2012). Of remark, *all of these cases,* either classical or novel ones, *are generally not "pure" blepharitis.* That's why some authors reserve the term "blepharitis" to subacute or chronic forms, where the process is actually confined to the lid margin (Duke-Elder and MacFaul, 1974; Brancato, 1978). Rather, in AB the lid margin is involved by a more extended process, not primarily interesting the lid margin itself, which becomes involved by contiguity. AB is typically associated with any type of acute keratoconjunctivitis or acute eyelid dermatitis, and stands out amid the extended differential of conditions inducing eyelid swelling (Ricketti et al., 2012). The association of recidivant blepharitis and keratitis in children can be erroneously attributed to staphylococci, whereas the correct diagnosis is herpes simplex infection (Liu et al., 2012). Other clinical clues can point to etiological diagnosis (e.g., *angular blepharitis* associated with angular conjunctivitis of *Moraxella* infection [Duke-Elder and MacFaul, 1974], which can complicate steroid therapy, leprosy, diabetes mellitus, varicella-zoster infections, protein malnutrition, and can involve the cornea and the sclera [Garg et al., 1999]). In some cases the extension process would not be metastatic; rather, it could represent an example of the neglected concept of *contiguous inflammation*, which gastroenterologists (Grucela and Steinhagen, 2009), and possibly laymen, are more familial with than ophthalmologists (Goldberg et al., 1989) and dermatologists (Helmbold et al., 1999). This term refers to an unspecific extension of inflammation to adjacent tissues through diffusion of mediators and migration of inflammatory cells. However, even in apparently trivial cases, the application of this concept must not be abused, because *specific* pathologic processes can develop as a consequence of the underlying disease. For instance, severe ulcerative blepharitis with involvement of follicles of lashes developing in patients with atopic dermatitis can be the expression of a *Candida* infection. These cases of severe recalcitrant "atopic blepharitis", which worsens in correspondence with flare-ups of the cutaneous disease, require repeated scrapings and culture (Huber-Spitzy et al., 1992). Less severe, but similar cases, with redness, itching of the margin of the eyelids, and microulcerations seem to be caused by fungi of the genus *Malassezia* (Derbel et al., 2005).

Table 1. Causes of acute blepharitis

Causes
Bacterial infections (*Staphylococcus aureus, Moraxella* spp., others, even specific - trachoma)
Mycotic infections (*Pityrosporum* [*Malassezia*] spp., *Candida* spp., opportunistic fungi in immunocompromised patients)
Parasitic infestations (mainly *Phthirus pubis*; arthropod assaults)
Viral infections (*Herpes simplex, Herpes zoster*, several viral infections, with and without exanthema)
Dermatitis of the eyelid (atopic, contact allergic, irritative)
Drug allergy (exhaustive list in [Hampton Roy, 1993]; erythema multiforme major and Stevens-Johnson syndrome)
Nutritional deficiencies (biotin, vitamin B_2, zinc)
Local trauma (rubbing, foreign body, photoexposition, pollutants)
Contiguous inflammation from adjacent inflamed sites

Exhaustive lists and discussions of concomitant, favoring, or associated etiological factors are well represented in classical textbooks (Duke-Elder and MacFaul, 1974; Trevor-Roper, 1974; Toselli and Miglior, 1979; Hampton Roy, 1993), and sometimes they are worthwhile to be browsed through with a "brute force" approach to differential diagnosis (Table 1). However, before embarking upon such a time-consuming and expensive enterprise, a *clinical examination of the whole integument and accessible mucosae* is mandatory.

Sometimes this leads straightforward to correct diagnoses such as trivial atopic dermatitis, but also clinical overture of *erythema multiforme major* or *Stevens-Johnson syndrome, acrodermatitis enteropathica* (Azemi et al., 2012), *ariboflavinosis (vitamin B_2 deficiency), biotinidase deficiency* (Rajendiran and Sampath, 2011), and *xeroderma pigmentosum* (Brooks et al., 2013). It is glooming to state that such a simple procedure is often omitted - not only by ophthalmologists!

Acute Blepharitis: What Dermatologists Should Do?

Even if the diagnosis is straightforward (contiguous inflammation from or specific extension to the margin of the eyelid of primarily dermatological disease of the lid itself), proceed to a complete (i.e., naked patient) inspection of the skin. Obtain a complete drug and allergy history. Make use of Wood's lamp to track louse nites down. Refer to the ophthalmologist, require proper labs, including scraping and cultures whenever indicated. Specify the suspicion for unusual infections, and ask for appropriate examinations (culture on special media, PCR).

2. Chronic Blepharitis: Always Recalcitrant

When AB *of any etiology* has settled down, or, quite more often, since its very beginning, blepharitis can be *chronic* (CB). This means a low intensity, spoiling, continuous, dull disease which threatens often severely the chances of a good quality of life of affected people, and sometimes has ominous implications as to the visual function, such as corneal alterations, neovascularization and pannus formation. In anterior forms, eyelashes can be definitively lost, and the eyelid margin can be thickened and deformed by the scarring process (Duke-Elder and MacFaul, 1974). It appears to be rare – or probably underrecognized, even in the absence of slit lamp examination – in dermatological practice, but can account for up to 47% of diagnoses in ophthalmologic settings, where it stands out as the most frequently diagnosed condition (Craig, 2013). The complexity of the lid margin (folliculoglandular structure) favors the chronicization, in form of CB, of any dermatitis involving the eyelids, even when this is healed or in remission as to the skin side (Duke-Elder and MacFaul, 1974). Thus we must admit that CB can ensue from dermatologists' faults of postponement and irresolution.

2.1. Classification of Chronic Blepharitis: Topographic versus Pathologic

The evolution of the nosographic concept of CB has been disappointing over decades, and current classifications are cause of confusion, because of overlaps, cumbersome terminology, and "more probably, because the pathogenesis is very poorly understood with few unifying concepts" (Leonard and Dart, 2010). Two topographic forms (Table 2) are recognized: *anterior* CB, where the pathologic process ensues from the lashes and their follicles; and *posterior* CB, which is pivoted on meibomian gland dysfunctions. Pathological classifications are descriptive, and distinguish (McCulley et al., 1982; Auw-Haedrich and Reinhard, 2007; Table 2):

- *Seborrheic/staphylococcal CB,* characterized by redness of the lid margin, and collarets of fibrinous secretion enveloping white or yellow scales. When the seborrheic component prevails, erythema is scanty, and the clinical picture is dominated by dry or greasy scales and secretion. This form could coincide with the *squamous type* of the historical, but not outdated, classification proposed by Thygeson (McCulley and Shine, 2000). The superimposition of Gram-positive agents, especially *Staphylococcus aureus, Propionibacterium acnes* and coagulase-negative staphylococci (Hoyt and Lambert, 1990), but possibly also *Malassezia* fungi (Derbel et al., 2005), enhances inflammatory phenomena, with pustular folliculitis of the eyelids leading to the formation of small ulcers (Thygeson's *ulcerative type* [McCulley and Shine, 2000]; *"acne blepharitis"* [Duke-Elder and MacFaul, 1974]). If the process is protracted, madarosis (loss of eyelashes) and trichiasis (inward turning of the eyelashes, which can scrap and injure cornea) can ensue. Seborrheic forms are more typical of adults, often with associated cutaneous seborrheic dermatitis, whilst staphylococcal CB, often starting as AB, is more common in younger people, including children (Turnbull and Mayfield, 2012; Hoyt and Lambert, 1990). Dripping of cocci through the nasolachrymal duct leads to chronic colonization of nostrils, and even to chronic staphylococcal infection of the face (sycosis of the beard of adults formerly affected by pediatric CB), from which staphylococci can be reimported to the eyelids (Duke-Elder and MacFaul, 1974).

Caveat for dermatologists: This classification can be misleading, since, in atopic or seborrheic patients, pustular/ulcerative folliculitis of the eyelashes can be related to Candida infection or to Malassezia, respectively, and not to Gram-positive cocci, as pointed out above. Refer to the ophthalmologist with an explicit request for swabs and specialized culture!

- *CB associated with meibomian gland dysfunction (MGD* [Table 3]*):* this presents with swelling and erythema of the internal border of the eyelid, coupled with thickening of the meibomian secretion ("meibum"), which becomes sticky and obstruct the meibomian ducts, and can sometimes be expressed with a toothpaste appearance. The gland duct orifices jut out (so called "pouting"), and are filled with the sticky secrete (Auw-Haedrich and Reinhard, 2007). These modifications lead to the formation of an abnormal tear film, with enhanced evaporative losses and chronic drying of the eyes (see Paragraph 2.2). Moreover, if damaged, obstructed meibomian ducts break down, their content leaks in the interstitium, leading to the formation of granulomatous lesions known as *chalazia*. These patients almost uniformly complain of dry eyes – and we'll see why (paragraph 2.2). Worthy of note, dermatologists can *cause* keratoconjunctivitis and CB with MGD when they prescribe *systemic isotretinoin* (Lebowitz and Berson, 1988). This drug is secreted by the lachrymal glands, thus affecting directly the anterior segment (Rismondo and Ubels, 1987). This kind of MGD seems reversible with discontinuation of the drug (Bozkurt et al., 2002). Similar considerations apply to *systemic acitretin* (Denis et al., 1993). The matter becomes peculiarly delicate and double-edged when isotretinoin treatment is warranted for severe papulopustular rosacea with ocular invovement. Other agents implicated in MGD are the *Epidermal Growth Factor inhibitors* (EGFi), included in various regimens for treatment of solid tumors (Borkar et al., 2013).
- *Mixed CB:* A substantial identity between anterior CB and seborrheic-staphylococcal CB, and between posterior CB and MGD-associated CB can be assumed for our purposes. When both coexist – and this is quite frequent, we speak of mixed CB. After having read paragraph 2.2, readers will agree that anterior CB is potentially or actually "mixed", because MGD is present in any form of CB, at least latently.
- *Infiltrating CB*: this is a "dermatological" addition that the author wishes to introduce. In this setting, the descriptive term "CB" is taken

literally at its facial value, i.e., without the specific nosographic and pathophysiologic connotations exposed above. The adjective refers to the progressive development of thickening and induration of the eyelid margin. Apart from *multiple chalazia*, a classical, specific form of CB is within dermatologists' province: this is *discoid lupus erythematosus (DLE) blepharitis.* It can remain undiagnosed for years (Huey et al., 1983), attains mainly the outer third of the inferior eyelid, and can extend to the whole eyelid (Panse et al., 2004). DLE-CB can cause considerable local damage, with madarosis and cicatricial ectropion, is itself associated with MGD (Kopsachilis et al., 2013) – thus secondarily complying with the specific concept of CB, and *can be unilateral* (Panse et al., 2004), a fact which exposes to considerable diagnostic hazard.

Table 2. Classification of chronic blepharitis: a practical correlation

Topographic:	*Pathologic:*
- Anterior	- Seborrheic/Staphylococcal (but also Fungine)
- Posterior	- Meibomian gland dysfunction (MGD)
- Whole margin of eyelid	- Mixed ("conjunctivalization" of lid margin)
- Unilateral	- Infiltrative (often false blepharitis: beware of malignancy)

Table 3. Meibomian gland dysfunction (MGD)

- Plane gland insufficiency (example: anihidrotic ectodermal dysplasia; gland surgical or inflammatory destruction; partial insufficiency: systemic retinoids)

- Meibomitis (examples: rosacea, seborrheic dermatitis), leading to:
    - Chemically and rheologically inadequate secretion
    - Obstruction of ducta
    - Loss of local defence / Bacterial overgrowth

- Loss of contact of gland ostia with the conjunctiva – "conjunctivalization" of the lid margin (examples: dermatological diseases involving the eyelid; ectropion of any cause)

Caveat for Dermatologists: False Infiltrative CB!

Blepharitis of any kind, either AB or CB, can start unilaterally, but invariably (with the exceptions of abortive forms, herpes infections, local trauma, and arthropod assaults) will become bilateral. The development of persistently unilateral, infiltrative recalcitrant CB, even in the setting of recurrent chalazia, should always raise the suspicion of *adnexal lid carcinoma* (the "monocle syndrome"), and prompt the clinician to send the patient for lid biopsy! On histological examination these cases could turn out to be *sebaceous carcinoma of Zeis's or meibomian glands*, or *signet ring-cell carcinoma* (Tanboom et al., 2013). Mistrust accommodation clinical diagnoses such as "chronic stye/hordeolum" or "anterior/external chalazion" as well: *basal cell carcinoma of the eyelid margin* is constantly in ambush, and timely diagnosis is mandatory.

Otherwise, the differential of infiltrative CB can include *cutaneous sarcoidosis* and *cutaneous lymphoma* (Ena et al., 2006), as well as the peculiar translucid "bead papules" of *blepharosis moniliformis*, the eyelid involvement of *lipoid proteinosis (Urbach-Wiethe disease* [Blodi et al., 1960]*)*. Once again, a thorough clinical and patological evaluation decides easily.

2.2. Chronic Blepharitis at Work: The Unfortunate Complementarity of Heterogeneous Mechanisms of Disease

This review is intended for practical clinicians: sophisticated results of basic research about pathogenesis of CB are beyond its scope, and the reader is referred to specific sources (McCulley and Shine, 2000; Auw-Haedrich and Reinhard, 2007). However, some basic concepts are of concern to the practical clinician, and cannot be omitted, especially in the perspective of rational treatment choices.

Classically (Duke-Elder and MacFaul, 1974), minor cases of anterior CB ensue in the settings of chronic exposition to local irritating noxae such as wind, smoke, sun, refractive errors (especially astigmatism and hypermetropia [Brancato, 1978]), strabismus, visual efforts in condition of poor lighting – and all of these factors must not go neglected. In the author's experience, frequent fliers are particularly at risk for minor spoiling forms of CB, maybe because of continual exposition to air-conditioning. Precipitating factors are represented by allergens, irritants (cosmetics, contact lenses [Khaireddin, 2013], and air pollutants [Malerbi et al., 2012]), reactivation of concomitant dermatological diseases involving the eyelids, or bacterial superimposition (see below). But, on the posterior side, why and how should meibomian glands "dysfunction"? In his seminal paper on CB, Thygeson observed that "infection of the meibomian glands is the greatest single factor that must be overcome.

Meibomianitis was present in all cases in which blepharitis was resistant to therapy" (McCulley and Shine, 2000). Not fortuitously, the classical example of MGD is represented by *rosacea,* whereas, albeit quite seldom, *ectodermic dysplasia* (Auw-Haedrich and Reinhard, 2007) would fit even more (complete failure of meibomian gland function). Retinoid intoxication provides a reversible experimental model of the process (see above), whereas dry eye and blepharitis are typical permanent outcomes of radiotherapy of the ocular region (Paik et al., 2012). Note that CB of any origin can lead by itself to loss of meibomian glands (Auw-Haedrich and Reinhard, 2007).

Taking rosacea as a model, it has been known for decades that meibomitis (the usual synonymous for meibomianitis) is frequent in rosacea patients, possibly due to the putative primarily inflammatory nature of this disease (Stone and Chodosh, 2004). MGD ensues, and the alterations in meibum secretion and composition lead to formation of an unstable tear film, drying of the eye, and bacterial superimposition with ocular surface inflammation, possibly favored by the activation of overexpressed bacterial lipases, especially staphylococcal ones. This process could be enhanced by elevated facial skin temperature in rosacea patients. Bacterial lipases further cleave meibum lipids, thus worsening the quality of the secretion itself and producing local proinflammatory substances, such as diglycerides and free fatty acids (Stone and Chodosh, 2004). But don't believe seborrheic blepharitis is solely anterior! Indeed, meibomitis is associated with this condition, too, and not only because of backward extension of the inflammatory process. The meibomian seborrhea (Culley et al., 1982) characterizing this condition, leads to a dysfunctional result similar to that of inflammatory MGD.

At this point we have gathered all sufficient data in order to track …

The first vicious circle in CB physiopathology (inner-outer): Primary inflammation/Dysfunction of meibomian glands → Tear film defect → Dry eye → Bacterial superimposition → Anterior extension of the process & Further worsening of lachrymal secretion → Intercurrent AB → Worsening of CB … *[start again and again → secondary blepharokeratoconjunctivitis; permanent corneal and lid scarring]*

Can this vicious circle work in a reverse form? Above, we asked ourselves why meibomian glands should dysfunction, and we reckoned on rosacea as a model for primary MGD. The fact is that MGD can be *secondary to anterior processes extending towards the conjunctiva.* 100% of patients with seborrheic

CB and associated secondary meibomitis, and 82% of patients with seborrheic CB have seborrheic dermatitis, respectively (Auw-Haedrich and Reinhard, 2007). By the way, the disputed kinship between seborrheic dermatitis and psoriasis is evident also at the ocular level: patients with psoriatic arthritis can present CB and dry eye (Lima et al., 2012). It has been known for decades that many patients with psoriasis suffer from CB (Altomare and Capella, 1994). Contiguous inflammation can lead to diffusion of proinflammatory factors, and favors hyperkeratinization of meibomian excretory ducts, with gland involvement and ensuing MGD. In seborrheic dermatitis, primary abnormalities of meibum composition contribute to blocking of excretory ducts and boost the development of MGD. But this is not the end of the story. Apart from intrinsic MGD, an extrinsic one can be recognized: in skin diseases involving the lid margin, the mucocutaneous junction can migrate posteriorly, with retroplacement of the meibomian orifices (so called "conjunctivalization" of the lid margin) and consequent defective function of the glands, even in absence of duct obstruction (Bron et al., 2011a, b). Moreover, plenty of dermatological diseases (Duke-Elder and MacFaul, 1974) can cause *ectropion* (i.e., the eversion of lid margins): *erythroderma* of any origin *(psoriasis, cutaneous lymphoma, pityriasis rubra pilaris ...), erysipelas, epidermolysis bullosa, ichthyoses, Darier's disease, Stevens-Johnson syndrome, bullous autoimmune diseases.* In these cases, meibomian glands cannot work properly simply because they lose contact with the conjunctival sac, but the undesirable result is the same – the process is only faster, and often severe. The clinical picture is dominated by dermatogenic keratoconjunctivitis, and CB simply joins other, more evident sequelae. *Entropion* can lead to conjunctivalization of the margin all the same, e.g. in *trachoma* (Lucena et al., 2012).

The overall result is clearly …

The second vicious circle in CB physiopathology (outer-inner): Primary inflammation arising in the skin *or* Direct exogenous insult to the lid border ("trivial AB") → Posterior extension of the inflammatory process & Bacterial superimposition → Involvement of meibomian glands (MGD plus conjunctivalization of orifices) → Tear film defect → Dry eye → *[Here enter the first vicious cycle]* → … *[start again and again* → *secondary blepharokeratoconjunctivitis; permanent corneal and lid scarring]*

Now, let's make a *Gedankenexperiment*: hit a given stage of both vicious circles with a treatment putatively apt to interrupt the circle itself. Repeat this experiment, quiz yourself what you would do if… This exercise in self-examination will help you to develop the right mind in order to tackle the problem of blepharitis treatment.

3. What Should Dermatologists Do with All This Stuff? The Diagnosis and Treatment Challenge

3.1. Choose and Strike

Whilst the treatment of "pure" acute eyelid dermatitis/blepharitis is often straightforward (oral acyclovir for herpes infections, topical low potency corticosteroids or calcineurin inhibitors for atopic dermatitis or contact dermatitis, and so on), treatment of CB is often an exhausting, deceiving effort in taking under control a disease for which there is no "cure" (McCulley et al., 1982). This fact is well reflected by the current heterogeneous panoply of available treatments. Given the underlying complicate, intricate physiopathology we sketched above, it must indeed be recognized that every therapeutic approach tackles the process at a given level. Accordingly, a "divide and conquer" approach aimed at unbundling components related to dry eye, CB, and exogenous sources of eye irritation should be warranted (Gilbard, 1999), in order to choose the most suitable one. The "vicious circle approach" we dealt with in the above paragraph provides us with a fairly reliable rationale. It is commonplace to state that diagnosis comes before treatment; thus we have to assess (↔ means "mainly relating to"):

1) History of exposition to exogenous noxious factors ↔ AB, anterior CB;
2) Coexisting skin diseases, especially:

- Rosacea ↔ posterior CB;
- Seborrheic dermatitis ↔ anterior and posterior CB;
- Atopic dermatitis ↔ AB, anterior CB;
- Irritant and Allergic contact dermatitis ↔ AB, anterior CB;
- Skin infections and infestations of the lid region ↔ AB, anterior CB;
- Unilateral eyelid disease ↔ AB, CB, dangerous malignant mimickers;

3) Microbial flora and other biologic agents;
4) Topical dye staining tests and tear film function.

Although it is recommended to keep anterior and posterior CB distinct (Lindsley et al., 2012), such a stratification of patients is artificial in clinical practice: we have seen why. The "double vicious circle" approach implicitly includes both categories of patients, as well as any transition or merging between them.

Items 1 and 2:

These have been discussed in the above paragraphs. The importance of careful history and local inspection cannot be overrated. It goes without saying that *patch-testing* should be warranted in the suspicion of exposition to allergens. Specialized series reserved to patients wearing contact lenses include thimerosal, ethylendiaminotetraacetic acid, chlorexidine gluconate, benzalkonium chloride and phenylmercury nitrate, and are commercially available (Sertoli et al., 2003). Don't forget that these visual aids also increase the risk of bacterial blepharitis (Turnbull and Mayfield, 2012). As to seborrheic/squamous CB, classical prescriptions include removal of scales with warm compresses or baby shampoo, and this first-line approach is still recommended (Turnbull and Mayfield, 2012). Heating of meibomian glands could favor release of warmed oils from the gland, thus improving obstructive MGD, and an appropriate device, the Lipiflow® Thermal Pulsation System, has been approved for therapeutic use - possibly an hi-tech version of warm compress application, but not an easily available one (Craig, 2013). However, dermatologists dislike lid hygiene with shampoos, because of the risk of exacerbating inflammation when a nonspecific, aggressive product is applied to the periocular structures (Craig, 2013). In the setting of contact lens wearing-related CB, it has been demonstrated that more specifically formulated phospholipid-liposomal solutions, could be better than baby shampoos, because of their favourable substitutive effect with consistent improvement of tear break-up time and subjective symptoms (Khaireddin and Hueber, 2013). Gauze compresses imbued with poloxamer, Aloe vera, chamomile extract, and other akin devices (Guillon et al., 2012), are commercially available and less irritant than detergents. However, they are not cheap.

The following items imply strict collaboration between dermatologists and ophthalmologists, *whom patients with blepharitis of any kind must be referred to.* But how can the ophthalmologists' responses turn useful to dermatologists? Stay with us…

Item 3 – Microbial flora and other biologic agents:

Staphylococcus and *Propionibacterium* strains are typically cultured with traditional microbiological techniques (lid scrapings, swabs) from patients with blepharitis, along with other occasional organisms such as streptococci, *Proteus*, *Pseudomonas* and yeasts (Duke-Elder and MacFaul, 1974). However, many agents could escape this approach because they hardly grow on cultures. Accordingly, molecular biology studies on the microflora of the conjunctiva have been performed in order to overcome the troubles inherent in the culture-based approaches. In a recent Korean study (Lee et al., 2012), samples were represented by tears and epilated eyelashes. Bacterial 16S rRNA genes were analyzed, and results were surprising. Whilst confirming that *Staphylococcus* is more represented in samples from patients with blepharitis, and can act as a causative agent in conformity with traditional views, subjects with blepharitis seem to harbor less *Propionibacterium* than healthy ones, albeit this agent could play a role in MGD-related keratoconjunctivitis, possibly inducing a delayed type hypersensitivity response (Suzuki, 2012). Remarkably, the study revealed that blepharitis patients harbored plenty of *Enhydrobacter, Streptophyta,* and other agents, the main sources of which are plant pollens, dusts, and soil particles. Lee and coworkers thus speculate that human blepharitis might be induced by infestations of mixed skin microbial flora, as well as the quoted environmental “dirt” (Lee et al., 2012) – an highly sophisticated confirmation of old clinicians’ wisdom (see paragraph 2.1). On the other side, these authors dispute the role of *Demodex* mites *(D. folliculorum, D. brevis)*, which are historically recognised as etiological agents of CB (Duke-Elder and MacFaul, 1974). Dermatologists, too, are at odds as to the role played by *Demodex* in skin diseases, and especially in rosacea (Elston, 2010). The overrepresentation of *Demodex* in blepharitis could be an epiphenomenon of enhanced sebum secretion in these patients, which favours mite growth (Lee et al., 2012), whereas other authors purport that ”demodicosis may cause itchiness in the eyelids and cylindrical dandruff in the lash roots” (Kosik-Bogacka et al., 2012), an opinion supported by a recent metanalysis (Zhao et al., 2012). However, the controversy could settle down when faced at the fact that *Demodex* mites harbour the Gram-negative bacterium *Bacillus oleronius*, which, coupled with mites themselves, could act as a co-pathogen in the development of severe forms of blepharitis (Szkaradkiewicz et al., 2012). The *Demodex* question, so well addressed by Polish investigators as to CB (Czepita et al., 2007), could be perhaps summarized by Elston’s witticism: “It may not be a matter of ‘do you have mites’, but rather ‘are your mites ill’ ” (Elston, 2010). Strains of *B.oleronius* are sensitive to doxicycline, gentamycin, and ciprofloxacin (Szkaradkiewicz et al., 2012).

It should be easy for dermatologists to remember that fungi of the *Candida* or *Malassezia* genera, may be sporadically involved in acute blepharitis, especially in atopic or seborrheic patients, respectively.

Owing to the fact that specialized sampling and examination techniques are often unavailable, an empirical approach is needed. The tenet that an heterogeneous flora is represented in blepharitis, and the recognized role of *Staphylococcus* as well, has prompted clinicians to use a variety of antibiotic agents in CB. It must be stressed that sometimes even topical antibacterials can induce blepharitis (e.g., levofloxacin [Kanda et al., 2012]). Eye drops or eye ointments containing *tetracyclines, fluoroquinolones, aminoglycosides,* and *chloramphenicol* are the blockbusters. *Sulfacetamide* must not go forgotten (Fine and Arndt, 1985): it inhibits all bacterial strains empirically isolated from swabs of anterior eyes segment (Roth et al., 1992). However, sulfacetamide eyedrops can even induce toxic epidermal necrolysis, especially in subjects formerly exposed to sulfonamides (Byrom et al., 2013). In some countries, sulfacetamide is also marketed in combination with astringents such as nafazoline or zinc phenolsulphonate. Topical *bibrocathol* is commercially available, and seems to display either astringent or antiseptic properties (Bezdetko et al., 2012), which could act synergistically. Topical *azithromycin* has been tried as well (Fadlallah et al., 2012). The author, following others (Turnbull and Mayfield, 2012), often favors *fusidic acid,* otherwise neglected in spite of its anti-inflammatory properties, and advises dermatologists not to be afraid of ophthalmic drugs, and rather become knowledgeable with at least four different antibiotic eyedrop/eye ointment proprietary preparations, *given their substantial practical equivalence.* Indeed, results are often quite favourable, albeit short lived, because of induced resistant strains and the heterogeneity of the involved flora. When we instill tobramycin, we are not sure whether we are targeting staphylococci, *B. oleronius* – or something else. Moreover, the underlying processes remain unaffected by topical antibiotic treatments. On the contrary, this could be the case for *oral tetracyclines,* that are worthy in the treatment of rosacea and, by extension, of MGD of any origin. This is not only because of their antibiotic effect, but because they exert an anti-inflammatory action as well (Turnbull and Mayfield, 2012; see below, Item 4). Although not substantiated by controlled studies, observational experience purports the assertion that tetracyclins, but not macrolides (erythromycins), are effective in ocular rosacea. Unfortunately, tetracyclines are ordinarily contraindicated in childhood, but pediatric ocular rosacea has responded to systemic erythromycin (Miguel et al., 2012). For pediatric patients with severe blepharitis associated with conjunctivitis, other systemic antibiotics that have been evaluated include *coamoxiclav* (amoxicillin-clavulanate [Cehajic-Kapetanovic and Kwartz, 2010]) and *azithromycin* coupled with topical loteprednol or cyclosporine A eyedrops (Choi and Djalilian, 2013). The fact that antibiotics commonly used in acnes vulgaris prove effective could imply a favourable effect on *Propionibacterium acnes* present in meibum (Suzuki, 2012).

Demodex infestation can be addressed with *topical acaricides (lindane, permethrine)*, which unfortunately are often irritant when applied in the eyelid district. *Tea tree oil* (the extracted oil of *Melaleuca alternifolia*, which is allergizing by itself [Crawford et al., 2004]) has been proposed with good results (Kheirkhah A et al., 2007; Patel and Raju, 2013) apparently even in a randomized controlled trial (Koo et al., 2012), but the association of lid scrubbing does not allow really to appreciate the relative weight of either procedure, and casts the shadow of bias on the whole study. *Oral ivermectin,* which can be rationally combined with oral metronidazole (Abdel-Badie Salem et al., 2013) or topical permethrine (Damian and Rogers, 2003), is probably better, especially in the critical setting of immunocompromised patients with widespread infestation and eruptive chalazia (Damian and Rogers, 2003). However, in several countries ivermectin is still only for veterinary use.

To date and to the best of the author's knowledge, no antifungal eyedrop/eye ointment preparations are commercially available – just as it was pointed out in 2005 by Derbel and coworkers, who applied successfully *ketoconazole* cream in a case of *Malassezia* blepharitis (Derbel et al., 2005). Systemic antifungal agents of the azole group could be considered in selected cases on the ground of positive mycological isolates. The reduction of the mycotic burden is classically recognized of paramount importance in patients with seborrheic dermatitis and CB, and in this regard systemic therapy can be better than traditionally recommended topical one (Fine and Arndt, 1985).

Phthiriasis must be tracked (Wood's light is of great help to highlight nits glued to the eyelashes) and treated (ol' *Golden mercury ointment*, or any greasy preparation, which smother parasites and their eggs, work miracles). *Viral (HPV) warts* or *molluscum contagiosum ("water-warts")* of the eyelids must be recognized and treated, in that they act as local irritative and anatomy-distorting factors. Clearly, selected cases of involvement of the eyelid margin or of the conjunctiva must be referred to the eye surgeon.

Item 4 – Topical dye staining tests and tear film function:

The dry eye disease in typical CB is evaporative (i.e., lachrymal secretion is present, but is functionally defective [Cuevas et al., 2012], whilst other diseases, such as Sjögren syndrome, are characterized by insufficient tear secretion [Perry and Donnenfeld, 2004; Kaercher and Bron, 2008]). Accordingly, even "know-it-all" dermatologists' patients are obliged to seek ophthalmologic consultation in order to have their Schirmer's test and tear break-up time evaluated (BUT: the interval between a complete blink and the appearance of the first randomly distributed corneal dry spot after instillation of fluorescein. A reduced BUT indicates mucin-deficient tears [Kim, 2000]), along with rose Bengal or less toxic (Bron et al., 2003) lissamine green test to spot eye surface alterations (Kim, 2000; Bron et al. 2003; Bron et al., 2011a). Other specialized tests can be provided (Bron et al., 2003; Bron et al., 2011a; Cuevas et al., 2012), but these are time-consuming, expensive, and require dedicated facilities. Anyway, conventional tests are often sufficient to show relevant abnormalities of the tear meniscus, instable tear film, displacement of Marx's line (roughly and inaccurately, the border between conjunctiva and keratinized skin marked by lissamine green stain [Bron et al., 2011a]) or its variations of staining intensity, which is relevant as to the evaluation of MGD (Bron et al., 2011b). CB patients almost invariably display a host of lachrymal abnormalities, and this evidence intuitively prompts to prescribe "innocuous" *lubricating drops* ("artificial tears"), provided these preparations, which generally contain hydroxypropyl methylcellulose, carboxymethylcellulose, sodium hyaluronate and other polymeric viscosity agents (Wander and Koffler, 2009), do not contain also irritating or allergizing chemicals – but this often can be verified only on a case-per-case, proof-and-error ground. However, the implications of lachrymal dysfunction linked with MGD, coupled with evident inflammation of the lid margin and/or of the conjunctivae, have turned the attention of clinicians to the use of anti-inflammatory drugs. *Topical corticosteroids*, often in association with antibiotics, are time-honored and widely used as a first approach. Care must be taken when topical corticosteroids are used, either as eye preparations or dermatological ones applied to the eyelid district: dermatologists must be aware of ophthalmologic steroid adverse effects related to prolonged treatment (Auw-Haedrich and Reinhard, 2007), such as elevated intraocular pressure, cataract formation – as well as thinning of the eyelid skin, of course (Stone and Chodosh, 2004)! Accordingly, in recent years a breakthrough has come with introduction of *topical cyclosporine A (CyA, CsA)*. Available as a 0.05% active principle emulsion in an artificial tear vehicle, it is indicated in dry eye disease. As to MGD, it can favorably affect meibomitis, with benefit on plugging of ducts and overall improvement of gland function without the adverse effects of topical corticosteroids (Perry and Donnenfeld, 2004), and could prove useful in ocular rosacea (Stone and Chodosh, 2004). It would seem paradoxical that an immunosuppressant acts in a favourable way in a disease with potential infectious components – but not to dermatologists, who know well how cutaneous infections in patients with atopic dermatitis are reduced by application of the immunosuppressive tacrolimus, which restores the cutaneous barrier through reduction of inflammation. *Tacrolimus,* which shares the mechanism of action with CyA (inhibition of calcineurin), is commercially available as 0.03% and 0.1% ointment. Albeit intended for skin application, the standard 0.03% preparation appears tolerable and effective if applied in the conjunctival sac. This has been demonstrated by an off-label use, pilot study in patients with allergic conjunctivitis (Attas-Fox et al., 2008), whereas other authors applied the 0.1% preparation only to the eyelid skin of patients with severe atopic blepharitis (Mayer et al. 2001). The related compound *pimecrolimus*, available as a cream, has successfully been used in refractory severe CB without evidence of infection (Auw-Haedrich and Reinhard, 2007). Topical tacrolimus and pimecrolimus are indicated for eyelid skin rash and hyperemia due to EGFis used in the treatment of solid tumors (Borkar et al., 2013). Clearly, like corticosteroids, these immunosuppressive drugs are better used after exclusion or taking under control of an active infectious process. Many ophthalmologists seem unaware of their existence, and, on the ground of the available literature and experience, could enjoy suggestions from dermatologists. Mooreover, tacrolimus inhibits signaling in the *Gli*-1 oncogene pathway. The Gli-1 protein codified by this oncogene is overexpressed in keloids, but not in scars or in normal skin, and the application of tacrolimus anecdotally lead to marked improvement of keloid skin lesions (Kim et al., 2001). Nobody has yet speculated about a putative influence of topical calcineurin inhibitors on the formation of corneal pannus: in the author's opinion, the question could make sense.

There are no studies about the effect on CB of drugs commonly used in acne therapy, such as *adapalene* and *azelaic acid*, in spite of the role played by *Propionibacterium acnes* in CB pathogenesis. Notwithstanding, they have been taken in consideration, at least in a prospective, speculative fashion (McCulley and Shine, 2000). The same applies to the anti-inflammatory action of the flavonoids *resveratrol* and *silymarin* (McCulley and Shine, 2000). From a theoretical viewpoint, adapalene, a naphthoic acid derivative with retinoid activity, could exert a favourable "unplugging" or "uncorking" effect on hyperkeratinized meibomian ducts. From an analogic viewpoint, it can be remarked topical tretinoin was tried for squamous metaplasia of conjunctiva in dry eye disease from several etiologies, but the reversal of keratinization was not reflected by clinical improvement, and the drug itself caused blepharoconjunctivitis (Soong et al., 1988).

3.2. And Beyond the Eyelids?

> The ætiology of blepharitis is rarely simple.
>
> (Duke-Elder and MacFaul, 1974)

The former paragraph was entitled "Choose and Strike" – why? The therapeutic arsenal sketched above cannot obviously be used all at once, and single most important pathophysiological problems must be tracked and recognized in a given patient: a topical prescription overburden (antibiotic ointment and artificial tears and anti-inflammatory eyedrops and…) will invariably lead to bad compliance. Moreover, related futile medical expenses make such an approach unfair and even unethical. Though we have already dealt with some systemic treatments above, this is the place to stress that *systemic therapy has a role in CB, and must be exploited.* This can be done even on empirical basis, relying on the properties of *oral tetracyclines,* administered for 4-6 weeks at least, which improve the function of meibomian glands, and inhibit the bacterial lipases responsible for proinflammatory phenomena and the formation of dysfunctional secrete (see above, paragraph 2.2; McCulley and Shine, 2000; Auw-Haedrich and Reinhard, 2007). In children, erythromycins can work the same way, and have a topical steroid sparing effect (Auw-Haedrich and Reinhard, 2007). Of course, treatment with *hydroxychloroquine* and photoprotection is highly effective on the specific disease component of LED-CB (Panse et al., 2004; Kopsachilis et al., 2013), but the sequelae easily fall in the domain of ordinary CB. In critical cases, even pediatric ones, use of systemic immunosuppressant drugs (azathioprine, mofetil mycophenolate) can be warranted. A useful "therapeutic ladder" has recently been provided by British investigators (Hamada et al., 2012).

Environmental and hygienic measures are of paramount importance, but it must be admitted that they are often spoiling or impracticable. Steel workers suffer from blepharitis and other inflammatory diseases of the anterior segment of the eye twice than factory staff personnel not directly involved in the industrial process (Mel'nichenko et al., 2012). Protective eyeglasses are undoubtedly of help, but workers too often find them annoying. Don't forget correction of refractive errors: in Hong Kong, 86% of eyes of adult patients with Down syndrome were affected, and 44% presented with blepharitis and chalazion as well (Fong et al., 2013).

In other clinical settings, ocular manifestations including CB, are represented, but have no specific value as to the recognition of specific ocular inflammation associated with the underlying disease. Anyway, sometimes they respond to specific therapy for the underlying disease. This is the case of CB associated with *inflammatory bowel disease* (Cloché et al., 2013). From a more general viewpoint, it is classically suggested that medical chronic conditions such as *diabetes mellitus* or *gout* are predisposing factors for CB (Duke-Elder and MacFaul, 1974; Brancato, 1978) – a point that should not be neglected. The eversion of eyelids consequent to *Graves-Basedow diseases* (Dalrymple's sign [Toselli and Miglior, 1979]) must be recognized and lead to correct diagnosis. *Androgen deficiency* (Sullivan et al., 2002) or *androgen resistance* are known favouring factors of CB in women (Auw-Haedrich and Reinhard, 2007), as well as estrogen deprivation in patients assuming aromatase inhibitors (Turaka et al., 2013), and these notions can be therapeutically exploited in appropriate settings.

Dermatologists are – or should be – great internists! They should not neglect the possibility of interventions aimed to the definitive correction of underlying general diseases occasionally manifesting themselves at the eyelid level.

Exercise: Go back to paragraph 1, and revise potentially corrigible internistic causes of AB.

We have browsed through the variegate world of blepharitides from the viewpoint of the skin doctor. Albeit we have recognized that mere descriptive, anatomoclinic definitions of such processes display important limitations, we have also spotted MGD as the crucial point to be focused over, because here is the "funnel neck", the crucial alteration where independent or mutually influencing disease processes draw together. The dermatologist's task, *before and after the mandatory referral to the ophthalmologist,* is to timely recognize either gross or subtle skin conditions that can extend to or influence the course of the blepharitis itself, in order to prevent the evolution of the process to the critical point, to help the ophthalmologist and collaborate with him/her in the search of the most specific, and possibly resolutive treatment. It has been purported that there is no strong evidence supporting any treatments for blepharitis in use (Lindsley et al., 2012). We feel authorized to frankly point out that people frantic with Evidence Based Medicine will be never able to successfully treat CB. As we have abundantly seen, evidence in this field is mainly observational or even anecdotal, and practical conduct ensues from a wise, improvised combination of classical concepts and innovative basic science results extrapolated to clinical practice (some would speak of "translational medicine" or other high-sounding words). Timid physicians, or those who think the quality of medicine must be judged "on the basis of cost, outcome, and, to a lesser degree *[sic!]*, patient satisfaction" (Webster, 1995) will never achieve adequate results. Here, patient satisfaction is the primary goal to be pursued, and turns out to be a good surrogate endpoint measuring that objective outcomes of irreversible anatomic distortion or even visual loss are far from becoming measurable.

References

Abdel-Badie Salem D, El-shazly A, Nabih N, El-Bayoumy Y, Saleh S. Evaluation of the efficacy of oral ivermectin in comparison with ivermectin-metronidazole combined therapy in the treatment of ocular and skin lesions of Demodex folliculorum. *Int. J. Infect. Dis.* 2013; 17: e343-7.

Altomare GF, Capella GL. Localizzazioni insolite della psoriasi. *It Gen. Rev. Dermatol.* 1994; 31: 95-7.

Amano Y, Sugimoto Y, Sugita M. Ocular disorders due to eyelash extension. *Cornea* 2012; 31: 121-5.

Attas-Fox L, Barkana Y, Iskhakov V, Rayvich S, Gerber Y, Morad Y, Avni I, Zadok D. Topical tacrolimus 0.03% ointment for intractable allergic conjunctivitis: an open-label pilot study. *Curr. Eye Res.* 2008; 33: 545-9.

Auw-Haedrich C. Chronische Blepharitis. Pathogenese, klinischer Verlauf und therapeutische Ansätze. *Ophthalmologe* 2007; 104: 817-28.

Azemi M, Berisha M, Kolgeci S, Avdiu M, Hoxha-Kamberi T, Daka A. Acrodermatitis enteropathica. *Medicinski Arhiv* 2012; 66: 137-9.

Bezdetko PA, Sergienko N, Dyomin Y, Korol A, Nikitin N, Merzbacher M, Groß D, Kohnen R. Successful treatment of blepharitis with bibrocathol (Posiformin® 2 %). *Graefes Arch. Clin. Exp. Ophthalmol.* 2012; 250:1869–1875.

Blodi FC, Whinery RD, Hendricles CA. Lipoid proteinosis (Urbach-Wiethe) involving the lids. *Trans Am. Ophthalmol. Soc.* 1960; 58: 155-6.

Borkar DS, Lacouture M, Basti S. Spectrum of ocular toxicities from epidermal growth factor receptor inhibitors and their intermediate-term follow-up: a five-year review. *Support. Care Cancer* 2013; 21:1167–1174.

Bozkurt B, Irkec MT, Atakan N, Orhan M, Geyik PO. Lacrimal function and ocular complications in patients treated with systemic isotretinoin. *Eur. J. Ophthalmol.* 2002; 12: 173-6.

Brancato R. *Appunti Sinottici di Oculistica.* Padua: C.E.D.A.M., 1978.

Bron AJ,Evans VE,Smith JA. Grading of corneal and conjunctival staining in the context of other dry eye tests. *Cornea* 2003; 22: 640-50.

Bron AJ, Yokoi N, Gaffney EA, Tiffany JM. A solute gradient in the tear meniscus. I. A hypothesis to explain Marx's line. *Ocul. Surf.* 2011; 9: 70-91 (a).

Bron AJ, Yokoi N, Gaffney EA, Tiffany JM. A solute gradient in the tear meniscus. II. Implications for lid margin disease, including meibomian gland dysfunction. *Ocul. Surf.* 2011; 9: 92-7 (b).

Brooks BP, Thompson AH, Bishop RJ, Clayton JA, Chan CC, Tsilou ET, Zein WM, Tamura D, Khan SG, Ueda T, Boyle J, Oh KS, Imoto K, Inui H, Moriwaki SI, Emmert S, Iliff NT, Bradford P, DiGiovanna JJ, Kraemer KH. Ocular manifestations of xeroderma pigmentosum. Long-term follow-up highlights the role of DNA repair in protection from sun damage. *Ophthalmology* 2013;120:1324-1336.

Byrom L, Zappalà T, Muir J. Toxic epidermal necrolysis caused by over the counter eyedrops. *Australas J. Dermatol.* 2013; 54: 144-6.

Cehajic-Kapetanovic J, Kwartz J. Augmentin duo in the treatment of childhood blepharokeratoconjunctivitis. *J. Ped Ophthalmol. Strab* 2010; 47: 356-60.

Choi DS, Djalilian A. Oral azithromycin combined with topical anti-inflammatory agents in the treatment of blepharokeratoconjunctivitis in children. *J. A.A.P.O.S.* 2013;17:112-113.

Cloché V, Buisson A, Tréchot F, Batta B, Locatelli A, Favel C, Premy S, Collet-Fenetrier B, Fréling E, Lopez A, Massoure MP, Humbert AL, Hansmannel F, Guéant JL, Bigard MA, Peyrin-Biroulet L, Angioi K. Ocular symptoms are not predictive of ophthalmologic inflammation in inflammatory bowel disease. *Dig. Liver Dis.* 2013; 45:

Craig JP. More than scratching the surface: a shift of focus in blepharitis management. *Cl. Exp. Ophthalmol.* 2013; 41: 522-3.

Crawford GH, Sciacca JR, James WD. Tea tree oil: cutaneous effects of the extracted oil of Melaleuca alternifolia. *Dermatitis* 2004; 15: 59-66.

Cuevas M, González-García MJ, Castellanos E, Quispaya R, de la Parra P, Fernández I, Calonge M. Correlations among symptoms, signs, and clinical tests in evaporative-type dry eye disease caused by meibomian gland dysfunction (MGD). *Curr. Eye Res.* 2012; 37: 855-63.

Czepita D, Kuzma-Grygiel W, Czepita M, Grobelny A. Demodex folliculorum and Demodex brevis as a cause of chronic marginal blepharitis. *Ann. Acad. Med. Stetin.* 2007; 53: 63-7.

Damian D, Rogers M. Demodex infestation in a child with leukaemia: treatment with ivermectin and permethrin. *Int. J. Dermatol.* 2003; 42: 724-6.

Denis P, Nordmann JP, Saïag P, Liotet S, Laroche L, Saraux H. Blépharo-conjonctivite chronique au cours d'un traitment par acitretine (Soriatane). *J. Franç. Ophthalmol.* 1993; 16: 191-4.

Derbel M, Benzina Z, Ghorbel I, Abdelmoula S, Makni F, Ayadi A, Feki J. Blépharite mycosique à Malassezia: à propos d'un cas. *J. Franç. Ophthalmol.* 2005; 28: 862-5.

Duke-Elder S, MacFaul PA. *The Ocular Adnexa – Part I, Diseases of the Eyelids* (volume XIII of the *System of Ophthalmology* edited by Sir S. Duke-Elder). London: Kimpton, 1974.

Elston DM. Demodex mites: facts and controversies. *Clin. Dermatol.* 2010; 28: 502-4.

Ena P, Pinna A, Carta F. Discoid lupus erythematosus of the eyelids associated with staphylococcal blepharitis and Meibomian gland dysfunction. *Clin. Exp. Dermatol.* 2006; 31: 77–79.

Fadlallah A, Rami HE, Fahd D, Dunia I, Bejjani R, Chlela E, Waked N, Jabbour E, Fahed S. Azithromycin 1,5% ophthalmic solution: efficacy and treatment modalities in chronic blepharitis. *Arq. Brasil. Oftalmol.* 2012; 75: 178-82.

Fine JD, Arndt KA. Seborrheic dermatitis. In: Demis DJ, editor. *Clinical Dermatology.* Twelfth revision. Philadelphia: Harper & Row; 1985. Volume 1: 1-7.

Fong AH, Shum J, Ng AL, Li KK, McGhee S, Wong D. Prevalence of ocular abnormalities in adults with Down syndrome in Hong Kong. *Br. J. Ophthalmol.* 2013; 97: 423-8.

Garg P, Mathur U, Athmanathan S, Rao GN. Treatrment outcome of Moraxella keratitis: our experience with 18 cases – a retrospective review. *Cornea* 1999; 18: 176-81.

Gilbard JP. Dry eye, blepharitis and chronic eye irritation: divide and conquer. *J. Ophth. Nursing Technol.* 1999; 18: 109-15.

Goldberg RA, Weisman JS, McFarland JE, Krauss HR, Hepler RS, Shorr N. Ocular inflammation and optic neuropathies associated with chronic sinusitis of intranasal cocaine abuse. Possible role of contiguous inflammation. *Arch. Ophthalmol.* 1989; 107: 831-5.

Grucela A, Steinhagen RM. Current surgical management of ulcerative colitis. *Mount Sinai J. Med.* 2009; 76: 606-12.

Guillon M, Maissa C, Wong S. Eyelid margin modification associated with eyelid hygiene in anterior blepharitis and meibomian gland dysfunction. *Eye Cont. Lens Sci. Clin. Pract.* 2012; 38: 319-25.

Hamada S, Khan I, Denniston AK, Rauz S. Childhood blepharokeratoconjunctivitis: characterising a severe phenotype in white adolescents. *Br. J. Ophthalmol.* 2012; 96: 949-55.

Hampton Roy F. *Ocular Differential Diagnosis*. Fifth edition. Philadelphia-London: Lea & Febiger; 1993.

Helmbold P, Kaufhold A, Hegemann B, Marsch WC. Contiguous inflammation of the skin. *Eur. J. Dermatol.* 1999; 9: 48-50.

Hoyt C, Lambert S. Lids. In: Taylor D, editor. *Pediatric Ophthalmology*. Boston-Oxford; Blackwell Scientific Publications; 1990; 141-55

Huber-Spitzy V, Bohler-Sommeregger K, Arocker-Mettingen E, Grabner G. Ulcerative blepharitis in atopic patients – is Candida species the causative agent? *Br. J. Ophthalmol.* 1992; 76: 272-4.

Huey C, Jakobiec FA, Iwamoto T, Kennedy R, Farmer ER, Green WR. Discoid lupus erythematosus of the eyelids. *Ophthalmology* 1983; 90: 1989-98.

Kaercher T, Bron AJ. Classification and diagnosis of dry eye. *Developm. Ophthalmol.* 2008; 41: 36-53.

Kanda Y, Kayama T, Okamoto S, Hashimoto M, Ishida C, Yanai T, Fukumoto M, Kunihiro E. Post-marketing surveillance of levofloxacin 0,5% ophthalmic solution for external ocular infections. *Drugs R.&D.* 2012; 12: 177-85.

Khaireddin R. Trockenes Auge bei Kontaktlinsenträgern. Aktuelle Studienergebnisse und ihre praktische Umsetzung. *Ophthalmologe* 2013; 110:511–514.

Khaireddin R, Hueber A. Lidrandhygiene bei Kontaktlinsenträgern mit Blepharitis. Therapievergleich Babyshampoo versus Phospholipidlösung. *Ophthalmologe* 2013; 110: 146-53.

Kheirkhah A, Casas V, Li W, Raju VK, Tseng SC. Corneal manifestations of ocular demodex infection. *Am. J. Ophthalmol.* 2007; 143: 743-9.

Kim A, DiCarlo J, Cohen C, McCall C, Johnson D, McAlpine B, Quinn AG, McLaughlin ER, Arbiser JL. Are keloids really "gli-loids"?: High-level expression of *gli*-1 oncogene in keloids. *J. Am. Acad. Dermatol.* 2001; 45: 707-11.

Kim J. The use of vital dyes in corneal disease. *Curr. Opin. Ophthalmol.* 2000, 11:241–7.

Koo H, Kim TH, Kim KW, Wee SW, Chun YS, Kim JC. Ocular surface discomfort and Demodex: effect of tea tree oil scrub in Demodex blepharitis. *J. Korean Med. Sci.* 2012; 27: 1574-9.

Kopsachilis N, Tsaousis KT, Tourtas T, Tsinopoulos IT. Severe chronic blepharitis and scarring ectropion associated with discoid lupus erythematosus. *Clin. Exp. Optom.* 2013; 96: 124–125.

Kosik-Bogacka DI, Lanocha N, Lanocha A, Crepita D, Grobelny A, Zdziarska B, Kalisinska E. Role of Demodex folliculorum in the pathogenesis of blepharitis. *Acta Ophthalmol.* 2012: e579 (doi: 10.1111/j.1755-3768.2012.02391.x; accessed March 26th, 2014).

Lebowitz MA, Berson DS. Ocular effects of oral retinoids. *J. Am. Acad. Dermatol.* 1988; 19: 209-11.

Lee SH, Oh DH, Jung JY, Kim JC, Jeon CO. Comparative ocular microbial communities in humans with and without blepharitis. *Invest. Ophthalmol. Vis. Sci.* 2012; 53: 5585-93.

Leonard JN, Dart JKG. The skin and the eyes. In: Burns T, Breathnach S, Cox N, Griffiths C, editors. *Rook's Textbook of Dermatology.* Eighth edition. Oxford-Chichester: Wiley-Blackwell; 2010: volume 4: 67.1-37.

Lima FB, Abalem MF, Ruiz DG, Gomez BdeA, Azevedo MN, Moraes HV Jr, Yeskel AS, Kara-Junior N. Prevalence of eye diseases in Brazilian patients with psoriatic arthritis. *Clinics (Saõ Paulo)* 2012; 67: 249-53.

Lindsley K, Matsumura S, Hatef E, Akpek EK. Interventions for chronic blepharitis. *Cochrane Database System Rev.* 2012: 5:CD005556 (accessed March 26th, 2014).

Liu S, Pavan-Langston D, Colby KA. Pediatric herpes simplex of the anterior segment. Characteristics, treatment, and outcomes. *Ophthalmology* 2012;119: 2003–2008.

Lucena A, Akaishi Santello PM, Rodrigues Veronesi MdL, Cruz Velasco AA. Upper eyelid entropion and dry eye in cicatricial tracoma without trichiasis. *Arq. Brasil. Oftalmol.* 2012; 75: 420-2.

Malerbi Korn F, Martins LC, Saldiva Nascimento PH, Braga Ferriera AL. Ambient levels of air pollution induce clinical worsening of blepharitis. *Environm. Res.* 2012; 112: 199-203.

Mayer K, Reinhard T, Reis A et al. 0,1% FK 506-Salbe - Eine neue therapeutische Option bei der atopischen Blepharitis. Klinische Studie an 14 Patienten. *Klin. Monatsbl. Augenheilkd.* 2001; 218: 733–736.

McCulley JP, Dougherty JM, Deneau DG. Classification of chronic blepharitis. *Ophthalmology* 1982; 89: 1173-80.

McCulley JP, Shine WE. Changing concepts in the diagnosis and management of blepharitis. *Cornea* 2000; 19: 650-8.

Mel'nichenko MA, Mal'tseva MB, Onishchenko AL, Lykova OF, Konysheva TB, Zabelin VI. [Chronic inflammatory and dystrophic diseases of the eye anterior segment and their association with genetic polymorphism in workers of metallurgic industry.] *Med. Tr. Prom. Ekol.* 2012; (6): 7-13 (Russian original; only English abstract retrievable).

Miguel AI, Salgado MB, Lisboa MS, Henriques S, Paiva MC, Cautela GP. Pediatric ocular rosacea: two cases. *Eur. J. Ophthalmol.* 2012; 22: 664-6.

Newell FW. *Ophthalmology. Principles and Concepts.* Fourth edition. Sant Louis: Mosby; 1978.

Paik JS, Cho WK, Lee SE, Choi BO, Jung SE, Park GS, Kim SH, Yang SW, Cho SG. Ophthalmologic outcomes after chemotherapy and/or radiotherapy in non-conjunctival ocular adnexal MALT lymphoma. *Ann. Hematol.* 2012; 91: 1393-401.

Panse I, Cordoliani F, Rybojad M, Rivet J, Lebbé C, Morel P. Blépharites du lupus érythémateux chronique. Quatre cas. *Ann. Dermatol. Vénéréol.* 2004; 131: 58-60.

Parkinson RW. Eyelid dermatitis. A common, often confounding rash. *Postgrad. Med.* 1996; 100: 231-6 (239-40).

Patel KJ, Raju VK. Ocular demodicosis. *West Virginia Med. J.* 2013; 109: 16-8.

Perry HD, Donnenfeld ED. Topical 0.05% cyclosporine in the treatment of dry eye. *Expert Opin. Pharamacother.* 2004; 5: 2099-107.

Rajendiran A, Sampath S. Biotinidase deficiency – clinching the diagnosis rapidly can make all the difference! *B.M.J. Case Reports* 2011; 2011 (doi:10.1136/bcr.07.2011.4494; accessed March 26th, 2014).

Ricketti AJ, Cleri DJ, Moser RL, Bilyk JR, Vernaleo JR, Unkle DW. A 44-year old man with bilateral eyelid swelling. *Allergy Asthma Proceed.* 2012; 33: 205-11.

Rismondo V, Ubels JL. Isotretinoin in lacrimal fluid and tears. *Arch. Ophthalmol.* 1987; 105: 416-20.

Roth HW, Leimbeck R, Sonnenschein B, Anger CB, Weber S. Zum antibakteriellen Wirkungsspektrum von Sulfacetamid. *Klin. Monatsbl. Augenheilk.* 1992; 200: 182-6.

Sertoli A, Ermini G, Pitonzo C. *Serie Standard (SS) e Serie Addizionali (SA) per la Diagnostica delle Dermatiti da Contatto.* Florence: F.I.R.M.A.; 2003.

Szkaradkiewicz A, Chudzicka-Strugała I, Karpiński TM, Goślińska-Pawłowska O, Tułecka T, Chudzicki W, Szkaradkiewicz AK, Zaba. Bacillus oleronius and Demodex mite infestation in patients with chronic blepharitis. *Clin. Microbiol. Infect.* 2012; 18: 1020–1025.

Soong HK, Martin NF, Wagoner MD, Alfonso E, Mandelbaum SH, Laibson PR, Smith RE, Udell I. Topical retinoid therapy for squamous metaplasia of various ocular surface disorders. A multicenter, placebo-controlled double-masked study. *Ophthalmology* 1988; 95: 1442-6.

Sullivan BD, Evans JE, Cermak JM, Krenzer KL. Dana MR. Sullivan DA. Complete androgen insensitivity syndrome. Effect on human Meibomian gland secretions. *Arch. Ophthalmol.* 2002; 120: 1689–1699.

Suzuki T. Meibomitis-related keratoconjunctivitis: implications and clinical significance of meibomian gland inflammation. *Cornea* 2012;31(Suppl. 1): S41–S44.

Tanboon J, Uiprasertkul M, Luemsamran P. Signet-ring cell/histiocytoid carcinoma of the eyelid: a case report and review of the literature. *Am. J. Dermatopathol.* 2013;35:e1–e5 (doi: 10.1097/DAD.0b013e318264991c; accessed May 26th, 1014).

Toselli C, Miglior M. *Oftalmologia Clinica.* Bologna: Monduzzi; 1979.

Trevor-Roper PD. *The Eye and its Disorders.* Third edition. Oxford-London: Blackwell Scientific Publications; 1974.

Turaka K, Nottage JM, Hammersmith KM, Nagra KP, Rapuano CJ. Dry eye in aromatase inhibitor users. *Cl. Exp. Ophthalmol.* 2013; 41: 239-43.

Turnbull AMJ, Mayfield MP. Blepharitis. *B.M.J.* 2012; 344: e3328 (doi: 10.1136/bmj.e3328; accessed March 26th, 2014).

Wander AH, Koffler BH. Extending the duration of tear film protection in dry eye syndrome: review and retrospective case series study of the hydroxypropyl cellulose ophthalmic insert. *Ocul. Surf.* 2009; 7: 154-72.

Webster GF. Is dermatology slipping into its Anec-dotage? *Arch. Dermatol.* 1995; 131: 149-50.

Zhao Ye, Wu LP, Hu L, Xu JR. Association of blepharitis with Demodex: a meta-analysis. *Ophthalm. Epidemiol.* 2012; 19: 95-102.

In: Conjunctivitis
Editor: Elias H. Bazile

ISBN: 978-1-63321-621-1

Chapter 2

INFECTIOUS CRISTALLINE KERATOPATHY

Valentín Huerva, MD, PhD, [*,1]**,**
Francisco J. Ascaso, MD, PhD [2]
and Jordi Soldevila, MD [3]

[1]Department of Ophthalmology, University Hospital Arnau de Vilanova, Lleida. Spain
[2]Department of Ophthalmology, Hospital Clínico Universitario "Lozano Blesa", Zaragoza, Spain
[3]Department of Ophthalmology, University Hospital Arnau de Vilanova, Lleida. Spain

ABSTRACT

Infectious crystalline keratopathy (ICK), first described in 1983, is a corneal infection characterized by branching, white, crystalline opacities within the corneal stroma and occasionally with anterior segment inflammation, with or without epithelial defect. Neither racial nor gender predisposition have been described. Risk factors for infectious crystalline keratopathy include long-term topical corticosteroid use, previous corneal surgery, prior corneal disease, systemic immunocompromised disorder and local anesthetic abuse. Diagnosis of ICK is basically established by clinical appearance on slit-lamp examination, but the isolation of

[*] Corresponding autor: Valentín Huerva, MD; PhD. Department of Ophthalmology, University Hospital Arnau de Vilanova, Lleida. Spain. E-mail: vhuerva@gmail.com

microorganisms may improve the effectiveness of treatment. It is not easy to isolate the agent, the infiltrate may often lie deep into the corneal stroma, and deep corneal scrapings or corneal biopsy may be required. Numerous microorganisms have been identified as causative agents, such as gram positive alpha hemolytic aerobic streptococcus (being the most common Streptoccocus viridans), staphylococcus (such as Staphiloccocus aureus and Haemolyticus), fungi, pseudomonas, mycobacterium, peptostreptococcus, corynebacterium, proprionobacterium and acanthamoeba. Differential diagnoses of ICK including fungal keratitis, bacterial keratitis, herpes simplex keratitis, graft rejection, Schnyder's dystrophy and multiple myeloma. First step treatment consists in topical antibiotics with bactericidal activity, such as vancomycin or other potent antibiotic agents with good gram-positive coverage, depending on culture or biopsy results. Response to medication is poor and slow because the bacteria are enveloped in a biofilm isolating the infectious organisms from the antimicrobial penetration. Some reports suggest the use of systemic antibiotics in severe cases. In absence of response antifungal therapy should be considered. Penetrating keratoplasty or lamellar keratectomy in patients with corneal scarring involving visual axis due to ICK may be helpful for visual rehabilitation.

Description

Crystalline keratopathy is a condition in which crystals are deposited in the corneal epithelium and/or in the anterior stroma. Affected individuals frequently are referred to the ophthalmologist with symptoms of pain, decreased vision or photofobia. This condition may arise from several causes, such as infection, corneal dystrophy or systemic disease, which result in a buildup of metabolic products in the cornea.

Infectious crystalline keratopathy (ICK) may occur with a bacterial infection. However other infectious agents may be present. The infection can arise de novo or as a sequelae of surgical procedures when the cornea is chemically or mechanically traumatized, such as refractive surgery and corneal transplants.

Infection-related crystalline deposits have fine branch-like shape or needle-like extensions in the corneal stroma resembling a snowflake; it develops over time and may be associated with inflammation. ICK is characterized by a white stromal infiltrate shaped branched fern, crystal-like, with integral epithelium and indolent course with or without a very discrete inflammatory reaction into the anterior chamber. Given the absence of suppuration and the presence of an integral corneal epithelium, this condition has been considered as an interstitial keratitis. No inflammatory reaction may be present in the areas of bacterial colonization [1, 2]. Although the most frequently agent which has been observed is the alpha-hemolytic streptococci, this condition can be produced by many species of aerobic and anaerobic bacteria [1-6].

Etiology

Even though ICK is most commonly associated with *Streptococcus* species (α-hemolytic *Streptococcus* is the most common cause), [2-6] this clinical entity may be caused by a variety of organisms. There are several case reports of clinical ICK from culture-proven Streptococcus *pneumoniae,* Staphylococcus epidermidis, *Haemophilus species, Enterocccus, Peptostreptococcus, Pseudomonas aeruginosa,* Acinetobacter, Citrobacter, Mycobacterium fortuitum, as well as *Candida Albicans, Alternaria,* fungi and Acanthamoeba among others [1-6]. Table 1 shows the possible infectious agents that may produce an ICK. It occurs more commonly in corneal grafts or otherwise immunocompromised corneas. The most common risk factors for ICK include history of penetrating keratoplasty (usually several months following corneal transplant), topical corticosteroid use, anesthetic drops abuse, contact lens wearing, trauma and systemic immunosuppression [2-9].

Pathogenesis

It is likely that gram-positive cocci from the periocular skin or conjunctiva gain access to the corneal stroma by tracking along suture lines or through micro-defects in the corneal epithelium. As opposed to many other bacterial infections of the cornea, the epithelium in IKC may appear intact and there is a paucity of inflammatory infiltrates [1, 2, 5]. Some authors have suggested bacterial colonies that cause ICK are less pathogenic, allowing them to invade and replicate within the stroma without inciting much response in the host. ICK seems to be mediated by the presence of a biofilm. Under certain circumstances, such as lack of nutrients [10], certain microorganisms are able to produce a biofilm, exopolysaccharides or matrix, which makes it difficult to eradicate germs due to masking of the antigens that involves a lack of immune response and the barrier effect motivates biofilm antimicrobial resistance in vivo [11-12]. A biofilm is a functional consortium of microorganisms organized within an extensive exopolymer matrix.

Table I. Infectious isolated agents in diagnosed cases of ICK

Bacteria	
Gram-positive	*Gram-negative*
Streptococcus Viridians Pneumoniae	Pseudomonas aeruginosa Pseudomonas fluorescens
Staphylococcus S.Aureus S.Haemolyticus S.Epidermidis	Haemophilus
Enterococcus	Acinetobacter lwoffi
Peptostreptococcus	Citrobacter koseri
Propionibacterium	Enterobacter aerogenes
Gemella haemolysans	Stenotrophomonas maltophilia
Corynebacterium	
Mycobacteria	
Mycobacterium Fortuitum	
Fungus	
Candida Albicans	
Alternaria fungi	
Protozoa	
Acanthamoeba	

Organisms within a biofilm are difficult to be eradicated by conventional antimicrobial therapy and can cause indolent infections [11].

Under certain environmental conditions such as nutrient limitation, some bacteria may secrete and reside in an exopolysaccharide glycocalyx polymer. This confers relative protection from humoral and cellular immunity, antibiotics and surfactants. Biofilms occur in natural aquatic ecosystems, on ship hulls, in pipelines and on the surface of biomaterials. They cause clinical infections of prosthetic hip joints, heart valves and catheters. Biofilm formation may occur rapidly on contact lenses and their cases and hence contribute to the pathogenesis of ICK. Bacteria within biofilms are 20-1000 times less sensitive to antibiotic than free-living planktonic organisms.

Existing experimental methods for modifying biofilm include the use of macrolide antibiotics that specifically impair biofilm production and the use of enzymes to digest it. These may have clinical applications, as potential adjunctive therapies to antibiotic therapy, for these resistant infections. Biofilm is an important cause of infections associated with biomaterials. Its formation occurs in ICK but probably not in chronic bacterial keratitis without crystalline changes. Secretion of an extracellular matrix by bacteria to constitute a biofilm is response to a nutrient-deprived environment in which growth and replication is depressed. The extracellular matrix of the biofilm may mask bacterial antigens, explaining the relative lack of inflammatory response in these infections. It may also be one of the mechanisms which explain the resistance to in vivo antimicrobial therapy when in vitro sensitivities have been proven [8, 12].

Clinical Symptoms and Signs

Gorovoy et al., [1] were the first on reporting a case of a crystal-like deposition associated with infection in the 80's as a unique and distinctive clinical entity characterized by white, branching, crystalline, opacities within the corneal stroma no associated with inflammatory response in a corneal graft. Since the first description various cases associated with different microorganisms were reported [2,13-15]. A sharply demarcated, snowflake-like stromal opacity on a background of clear, uninflammed corneal graft is the classic presentation (Figures 1,2 and 3), although variations on this theme are common [8, 9]. Visual loss is referred if the visual axis is affected. In some occasions an inflammatory reaction into the anterior chamber may be present [9]. Generally, the process is indolent.

Diagnosis

Diagnosis of ICK is basically established by clinical appearance on slit-lamp examination. Figures 1, 2, and 3 show different clinical aspects in the biomicroscopy of cases affected with ICK. Diagnostic testing such as gram stains, acid-fast stains, routine bacterial and fungal cultures, as well as mycobacterial cultures, should be obtained. It is important to realize, however, that culture yield may be low. In the first description, the crystalline appearance progressed over five months, and the patient eventually required a re-graft [1].

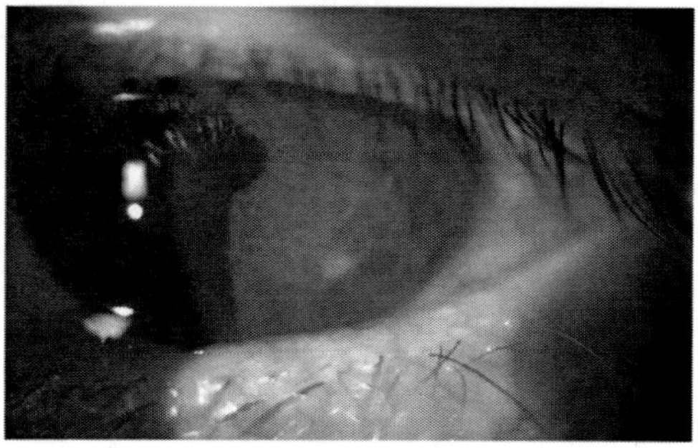

Figure 1. ICK with absence of response to topical antibiotics. Antifungal therapy improved the picture. ICK appeared after a corneal traumatism.

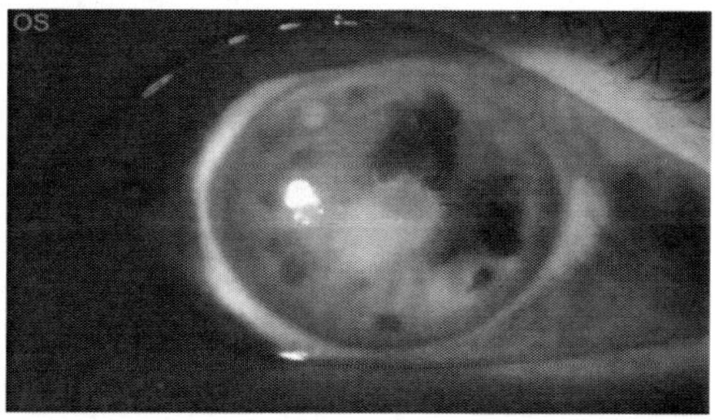

Figure 2. ICK by Enterococcus in a bandage contact lens wearer following vitreoretinal surgery (Adapted with permission from Lippincott Williams and Wilkins/Wolters Kluwer Health: Eye Contact Lens 2012; 38(1):72).

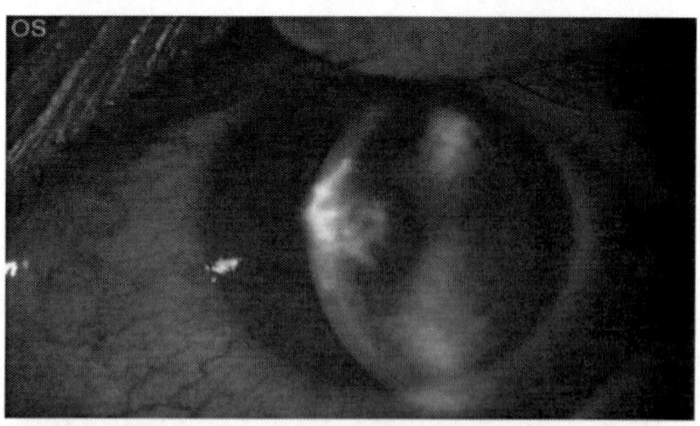

Figure 3. ICK by Pseudomonas fluorescens in a contact lens wearer (Adapted with permission from Lippincott Williams and Wilkins/Wolters Kluwer Health: Eye Contact Lens. 2013 Oct 9. [Epub ahead of print] PubMed PMID: 24113463).

There was no mention of any culture being performed, and no antibacterial therapy was given. Analysis of the corneal button removed showed a localized in growth of epithelium associated with a suture, and from this area colonies of Gram-positive bacteria were seen extending between the stromal lamellae. Though classic ICK is very distinctive, proper organism identification still requires isolation of the offending organism by deep corneal scrapings or corneal biopsy [6].

Histopathology of corneal biopsy or corneal buttons may reveal pockets of bacteria (usually Gram positive cocci) between intact lamellae of corneal stroma with a paucity of inflammatory infiltrate. The causative organism's agents have been previously enumerated. Eyes undergoing refractive surgery are at higher risk for infections with atypical organisms, such as mycobacteria (acid-fast bacteria) and *Alternaria* (fungi).

With the increasing number of patients undergoing refractive surgery and the relevance of early intervention, it is important to recognize ICK. It may also be seen in corneal grafts of eyes that have undergone penetrating keratoplasty and in those eyes that have an otherwise immunocompromised cornea (e.g., chronic corticosteroid use and topical anesthetic abuse). Histopathologic studies show a characteristic trilamellar structure of a bacterial cell membrane.

The organisms are present only anteriorly. Hematoxylin and eosin stains may reveal intrastromal pockets of basophilic material between the lamellae, with a notable absence of inflammatory cells. Gram's stain shows the basophilic material to be gram positive and transmission electron microscopy confirmed the presence of intrastromal pockets of bacteria.

The quite clinical appearance may make its infectious etiology unapparent [4]. Electron microscopy may show small electron-dense bodies with needle-like projectionis present. These bodies may be responsible for the crystalline appearance of this keratopathy [3, 5].

Differential Diagnosis

Differential diagnoses of ICK must be done with fungal and bacterial keratitis, herpes simplex keratitis, graft rejection, granular and Avellino corneal dystrophy, Schnyder's dystrophy and multiple myeloma.

Treatment

ICK management consists of steroids discontinuation and the administration of antibiotics. Unsolved infection, corneal scars or graft failure may occur, and transplantation is then required. [8] No significant differences in predisposing factors, clinical appearance, or visual outcomes have been described between infections caused by gram-negative bacteria and those caused by gram-positive bacteria.

After appropriate cultures, early and aggressive antibiotic therapy is mandatory. Treatment initially consists of cessation, or at least strict minimization, of topical steroids and prolonged use of topical antibiotics with bactericidal activity. Start with vancomycin, cefazolin or other potent antibiotic with good gram-positive coverage and adapting medications depending on culture or biopsy results are recommended [8, 9]. Systemic antibiotics are suggested in severe cases (9). In some occasions topical corticosteroids may be necessary if an inflammatory reaction into the anterior chamber is present [9]. However, ICK is notoriously difficult to treat, demonstrating poor and slow response to medications. Debilitating stromal scars or recurrence of infection are common. In many cases, despite appropriate antimicrobial therapy, repeated penetrating keratoplasty or lamellar keratectomy may be required.

When the organism has not been identified, a broad-spectrum antibiotic should be used [8, 9]. The antibiotic coverage should be tailored once the organism and antibiotic sensitivities have been obtained. If symptoms do not resolve, it is reasonable to expand coverage or to start systemic antibiotics. It is common for treating ICK to be necessary for weeks or even months. In cases that do not resolve after penetrating keratoplasty, the ophthalmologist may consider repeat surgical intervention as a last resort.

References

[1] Gorovoy MS, Stern GA, Hood CI, Allen C. Intrastromal non inflammatory bacterial colonization of a corneal graft. *Arch. Ophthalmol.* 1983;101(11):1749-52.

[2] Meisler DM, Langston RH, Naab TJ, Aaby AA, McMahon JT, Tubbs RR. Infectious crystalline keratopathy. *Am. J. Ophthalmol.* 1984 Mar;97(3):337-43.

[3] Samples JR, Baumgartner SD, Binder PS. Infectious crystalline keratopathy: an electron microscope analysis. *Cornea.* 1985-1986;4(2):118-26.

[4] Reiss GR, Campbell RJ, Bourne WM. Infectious crystalline keratopathy. *Surv. Ophthalmol.* 1986;31(1):69-72.

[5] Matoba AY, O'Brien TP, Wilhelmus KR, Jones DB. Infectious crystalline keratopathy due to Streptococcus pneumoniae. Possible association with serotype. *Ophthalmology.* 1994;101(6):1000-4.

[6] Khater TT, Jones DB, Wilhelmus KR. Infectious crystalline keratopathy caused by gram-negative bacteria. *Am. J. Ophthalmol.* 1997 Jul;124(1):19-23.

[7] Sharma N, Vajpayee RB, Pushker N, Vajpayee M. Infectious crystalline keratopathy. *CLAO J.* 2000;26(1):40-3.

[8] Huerva V, Espinet R, Ascaso FJ. Enterococcal infectious crystalline keratopathy in a wearer bandage contact lens. *Eye Contact Lens.* 2012; 38(1):72.

[9] Huerva V, Sanchez MC. Infectious Crystalline Keratopathy Caused by Pseudomonas fluorescens. Eye Contact Lens. 2013 Oct 9. [Epub ahead of print] *Pub. Med.* PMID: 24113463.

[10] Ormerod LD, Ruoff KL, Meisler DM, Wasson PJ, Kintner JC, Dunn SP, Lass JH, van de Rijn I. Infectious crystalline keratopathy. Role of nutritionally variant streptococci and other bacterial factors. *Ophthalmology.* 1991 Feb;98(2):159-69.

[11] Elder MJ, Stapleton F, Evans E, Dart JK. Biofilm-related infections in ophthalmology. Eye (Lond). 1995;9 (Pt 1):102-9.

[12] Fulcher TP, Dart JK, McLaughlin-Borlace L, Howes R, Matheson M, Cree I. Demonstration of biofilm in infectious crystalline keratopathy using ruthenium red and electron microscopy. *Ophthalmology.* 2001;108(6):1088-92.

[13] Dunn S, Maguen E, Rao NA. Noninflammatory bacterial infiltration of a corneal graft. *Cornea.* 1985-1986;4(3):189-93.

[14] James CB, McDonnell PJ, Falcon MG. Infectious crystalline keratopathy. *Br. J. Ophthalmol.* 1988;72(8):628-30.

[15] Tu EY, Joslin CE, Nijm LM, Feder RS, Jain S, Shoff ME. Polymicrobial keratitis: Acanthamoeba and infectious crystalline keratopathy. *Am. J. Ophthalmol.* 2009;148(1):13-19.

In: Conjunctivitis
Editor: Elias H. Bazile

ISBN: 978-1-63321-621-1

Chapter 3

AIR POLLUTION AND EMERGENCY DEPARTMENT VISITS FOR CONJUNCTIVITIS IN CALGARY, CANADA: A CASE CROSSOVER STUDY

Termeh Kousha[1,*] and Jessica Castner[2,†]
[1]Department of Mathematics and Statistics,
University of Ottawa, Ottawa, ON, Canada
[2]University at Buffalo School of Nursing,
Buffalo, New York, US

ABSTRACT

Objectives: Ambient air pollution exposure has been associated with the occurrence of several different health conditions.

These associations are not only limited to respiratory and cardiovascular system; there have been also number of studies that have linked ambient air pollutions to non-respiratory conditions, such as cardiac disease, appendicitis, headaches and migraines, skin conditions, eye discomfort and conjunctivitis. The purpose of this study was to

* Corresponding author: Dr. Termeh Kousha, Department of Mathematics and statistics, University Of Ottawa, 585 King Edward Ottawa, ON K1N 6N5. E-mail: tkousha@uottawa.ca.

† Jessica Castner: University at Buffalo School of Nursing, Buffalo, New York, US. E-mail: jcastner@buffalo.edu.

examine the associations between emergency department (ED) visits for conjunctivitis and ambient air pollution levels in Calgary, Alberta, Canada.

Materials and Methods: The National Ambulatory Care Reporting System was used to obtain patient information on ED visits for conjunctivitis for the period of January 2010 to December 2011. ED visits for conjunctivitis were defined using the International Classification of Diseases, Tenth revision (ICD-10) codes H10. A time stratified case-crossover design was applied in this study. Odds ratios (ORs) and their 95% confidence intervals (95%CI) for emergency department visits were calculated for one unit increase in each pollutant (nitrogen dioxide (NO_2), fine particulate matter with a median aerodynamic diameter of less than 2.5 μm ($PM_{2.5}$) and ozone (O_3)), controlling for temperature and relative humidity.

Results: Among 4,333 ED visits for conjunctivitis (49% females, 51 % males), analyses were conducted considering cold weather months (October to March) and warm weather months (April to September). During the warm months, statistically significant positive results were observed in the female population for NO_2 and for lags 5-7 days, with the highest result for lag 5 days (OR = 1.048; 95%CI = 1.020, 1.076) and in the male population for $PM_{2.5}$ lagged 6 days (OR = 1.014; 95%CI = 1.002, 1.026). During the cold months, statistically significant positive results were observed for females and NO_2 lagged 7 days (OR = 1.021; 95%CI = 1.001, 1.040) and for $PM_{2.5}$ for lag 2 days (OR = 1.042; 95%CI = 1.004, 1.079) and for males and O_3 lagged 5 and 6 days, with the highest result for lag 6 (OR = 1.035; 95%CI = 1.009, 1.062).

Conclusion: The findings of this study suggest that there are associations between level of air pollution and ED visits for conjunctivitis in Calgary, Canada. Our findings support associations reported in the literature for NO_2 among females. The latency period between exposure and ED visit for conjunctivitis in this study coincides with the typical incubation period for infectious conjunctivitis.

INTRODUCTION

Much of what is known about the etiology of conjunctivitis revolves around cellular microbiology, tissue pathology, and individual-level evidence [1, 2]. In the scope of socio-ecological concerns, this chapter describes the Socio-Ecological Model exemplifying the public-health policies and community-level factors linked to conjunctivitis.

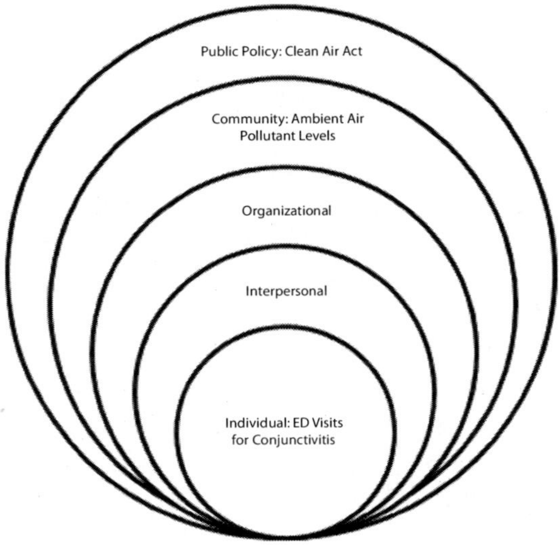

Figure 1. Socio-ecological Model for Ambient Air Pollutants and ED Visits for Conjunctivitis.

SOCIO-ECOLOGICAL MODEL

As depicted in Figure 1, human health is influenced by the interwoven influences of individual, interpersonal, organizational or institutional, communal, and public-policy factors [3, 4]. This study is pertinent to the public policies concerning clean air acts, to communal concerns about levels of air pollutants, and to individual health issues as the emergency department visits for conjunctivitis. While not addressed in this study, an example of interpersonal factor that impacts conjunctivitis may be caregiver's exposure to infected child, and an example of organizational factor would be a school policy on notifying parents about exposure to infectious conjunctivitis.

Public Policy Factors: Clean Air Acts

Public policies that may impact eye health include the development, monitoring, and enforcement of national clean air acts, and the related regulation intended to reduce emissions from common pollution sources like vehicles and industrial factories [5-7].

Public policy establishes levels that are considered safe and acceptable for human health [5] and selects pollutants for priority monitoring [7].

While many pollutants may impact eye health, only specific pollutants are routinely measured due to the current evidence of harm to human health, widespread nature of exposure, or exposure from multiple sources [6, 7].

The pollutants usually considered in the ecological air pollution studies include: ozone (O_3), nitrogen dioxide (NO_2) fine particulate matter (PM) with a median aerodynamic diameter of less than 2.5 μm ($PM_{2.5}$), carbon monoxide (CO), and sulfur dioxide (SO_2) [8-18]. Burning of fossil fuels is a common source for these pollutants; in particular, the combustion produces the automobile exhaust gases and most of the industrial emissions [19, 20].

Ground level ozone is generally created by sunlight acting on nitrogen oxides and other compounds.

As for the particulate matter, it may be composed of different types of organic and inorganic compounds, including compounds present in chemical emissions, in biologic material (pollens), or in dust from natural inorganic sources [6, 7].

Community Factor: Ambient Air Pollution

It has been confirmed that community ambient air pollution levels affect human health and are risk factors for respiratory conditions such as asthma [8, 9, 21-30] and also non-respiratory conditions, such as cardiac disease [9, 10], appendicitis [11], headaches and migraines [12], skin conditions [14-17], eye discomfort and conjunctivitis [17, 31-44].

While air pollution is linked to eye discomfort and conjunctivitis, the population burden for these disorders is understudied and underestimated.

Most of the direct cost and treatment for conjunctivitis are managed by patients and families through self-care and non-prescribed, over-the-counter products [45, 46].

Individual Factor: ED Visit for Conjunctivitis

Individual characteristics, such as gender and age, impact the risk of being affected by conjunctivitis [14, 47]. Both physiology and behavior can impact the risk [1].

ED visits, as a proxy for morbidity, provide a common individual-outcome measure in population studies [8-18]. The exact reason a patient chose to seek help in ED rather than try self-care or primary care, is often unknown. Since most conjunctivitis is treated at home with over the counter and self-care regimens, increased ED visits are likely due to symptom severity, increasing prevalence, or a combination of these factors [45]. It is plausible that even if there are no additional conjunctivitis cases in the population, an acutely worsening symptom severity leads patients to present the symptoms to the ED, also those who would normally self-manage the condition at home.

Alternatively, the exposure to the higher levels of air pollutants—as a biological stressor—may itself have enhanced the risk for the disease development, leading to higher frequency of ED visits. Finally, air pollutants such as particulates may deliver an infectious agent directly to the eye surface.

SETTING

The purpose of this paper was to investigate correlations between exposure to ambient air pollution and emergency department (ED) visits for conjunctivitis in Calgary, Alberta, Canada.

Calgary has the sunniest days year round of Canada's 100-largest cities, with just over 332 days of sun [48]. Calgary's altitude of over 1,000 meters above sea level is higher than the other North American settings where the relationships of air pollution and conjunctivitis have been studied [14, 47]. Strong west-winds dissipate the formation of low-level smog above the city. However, Calgary's growing population (as of the 2011 census, Calgary had a population more than a million, making it the largest city in Alberta), the increasing air emissions from vehicle travel, the road dust, and also the regional forest fires can cause air quality to deteriorate [48].

MATERIALS AND METHODS

Health Data

Data of ED visits for conjunctivitis were collected from hospitals in Calgary, Alberta, Canada. The visits were qualified using the International Classification of Diseases, Tenth revision (ICD-10) codes H10.

ED visit data for the period from January 2010 to December 2011 were retrieved from the National Ambulatory Care Reporting System (NACRS).

Broadly, the NACRS contains information collected at the time of healthcare service from participating hospitals, and includes information on day and night surgeries, outpatient clinics and ED data for all hospital community-based ambulatory care [49].

Environmental Data

Air pollution data were obtained from Environment Canada's National Air Pollution Surveillance Program (NAPS) [50]. Data from the NAPS stations located within 35 km distance from each patient's postal code were averaged. The data consisted of the daily average values of ozone (O_3), nitrogen dioxide (NO_2) and fine particulate matter (PM) with a median aerodynamic diameter of less than 2.5 μm ($PM_{2.5}$). Data for carbon monoxide and sulfur dioxide were incomplete; they were not included in the study.

Weather variables included the daily average temperature in degrees and the percentage of relative humidity; the daily data were calculated by averaging the hourly values. The data were retrieved from the Environment Canada stations located within 100 km of a patient's postal code and averaged if more than one station were located within the perimeter. Season was defined as cold weather months (October to March) and warm weather months (April to September). A dummy variable was created to represent season.

Statistics

A time stratified case-crossover (CC) design was applied [51]. The method was first introduced to epidemiology in 1991; presently it is commonly used in air pollution studies. The routine avoids confounding by patients' individual characteristics and slowly varying covariates (i.e., seasonal effects) [51-53]. A key feature of the CC design is using the cases that serve as their own controls: the control is the case in different time periods. Thus the control perfectly matches the case for the parameters other than environmental covariates.

A p-value less than 0.05 was considered statistically significant in all presented statistical results. The results are reported as odds ratios (ORs) and their 95% confidence intervals (CI).

ORs in the case of O_3, NO_2, and $PM_{2.5}$ were calculated by using the PROC PHREG procedure in SAS (Enterprise Guide, v.4.2). In the models, air pollutants and meteorological factors were lagged by the same number of days, from 0 to 8. For each case, three or four controls were created by making the case reappear on days matching the case's ED visit's day of week and month.

RESULTS

Figure 2 shows the number (counts) of conjunctivitis ED visits (N=4,333) by sex and age, from 0 years to 85 years of age. The patients of 85 years old age and older are represented on the graph as 98 years of age (i.e., by one point). Table 1 shows the number of ED visits stratified by sex, season, and ICD-10 code occurring in the period of January 2010 to December 2011. As one may see in Table 1, the majority of ED visits was qualified as "unspecified conjunctivitis" (ICD-10 code H10.9). The number of visits was higher during the warm seasons (61% of the total).

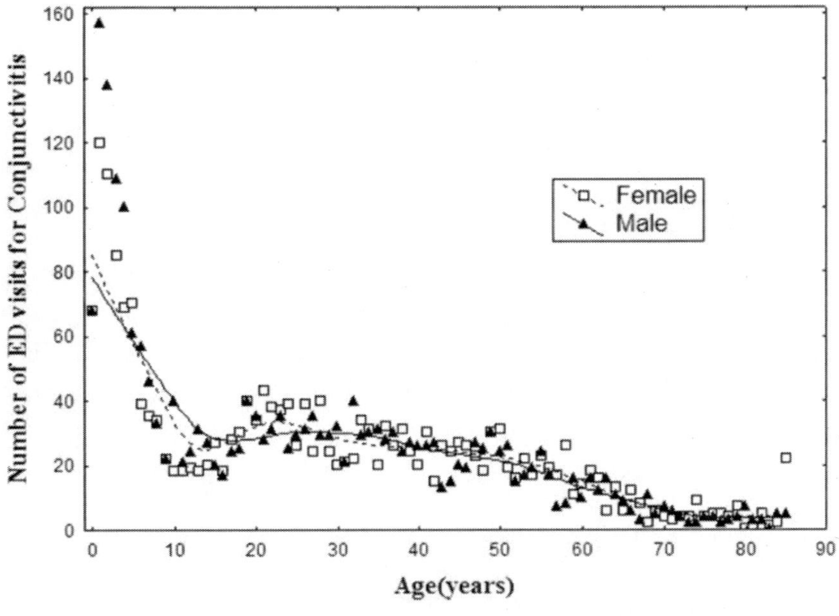

Figure 2. Frequency of ED visits for conjunctivitis by sex and age.

Table 1. Frequency of visits by sex, season (cold (October-March) and warm (April - September)) and by type (ICD-10 code)

	Frequency	%
Sex		
Female	2,113	49%
Male	2,220	51%
Season		
Cold	1,695	39%
Warm	2,638	61%
ICD-10 Code		
Mucopurulent (H10.0)	154	4%
Acute Atopic (H10.1)	479	11%
Other Acute (H10.2)	31	1%
Acute, Unspecified (H10.3)	210	5%
Chronic (H10.4)	6	<1%
Blepharoconjunctivitis (H10.5)	41	1%
Other (H10.8)	441	10%
Unspecified (H10.9)	2,971	69%
Total	4,333	

Table 2 characterises the relative humidity and temperature and gives descriptive air pollution statistics, for the city of Calgary.

Figure 3 shows estimated ORs and 95% CIs for ED visits for conjunctivitis in Calgary, Alberta, during the warm season. Statistically significant positive results were observed for the female population for NO_2 when applying lags 5-7 days, with the highest result obtained for lag 5 days (OR = 1.048; 95%CI = 1.018, 1.078). Also in the case of male population, for $PM_{2.5}$ lagged by 6 days, a significant result was obtained (OR = 1.013; 95%CI = 1.001, 1.026). In addition, there was a statistically significant negative result for males and NO_2 lagged by 4 days (OR = 0.962; 95%CI = 0.932, 0.992).

Figure 4 shows estimated ORs and 95% CIs for ED visits for conjunctivitis in Calgary, Alberta during the cold months. Statistically significant positive results were observed in the female stratum for NO_2 lagged by 7 days (OR = 1.020; 95%CI = 1.000, 1.040) and for $PM_{2.5}$ lagged by 2 days (OR = 1.041; 95% CI = 1.002, 1.081).

Also in the male stratum, for O_3 and lags 5 and 6 days, positive results occurred, with the highest result for lag 6 (OR = 1.035; 95% CI = 1.007, 1.062).

Table 2. Descriptive air pollution statistics and characteristics of relative humidity and temperature

City	Variable	Minimum	Mean	Maximum	IQR
Calgary	NO_2 (ppb)	1.4	15.0	47.0	11.8
	O_3 (ppb)	2.3	22.2	42.3	13.5
	$PM_{2.5}$ (ug/m3)	2.4	11.2	138.4	5.0
	Humidity (percentage)	16.1	63.0	99.4	24.8
	Temperature (Celsius)	-26.7	21.6	48.0	12.44

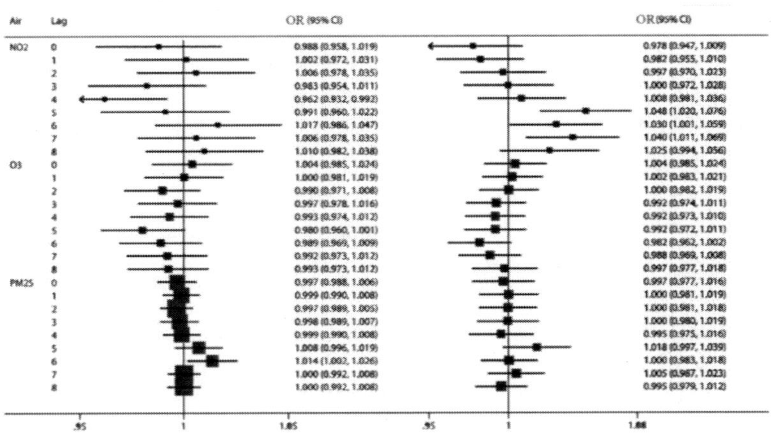

Figure 3. Results of fixed effect for conjunctivitis in Calgary during warm seasons.

Statistically significant negative results were observed for males and NO_2 at lag 6 days (OR = 0.972; 95%CI = 0.94, 0.996) and for $PM_{2.5}$ at lag 6 days (OR = 0.961, 95%CI = 0.925, 0.997).

Discussion

We investigated correlations between ambient air pollution exposure and ED visits for conjunctivitis, analysing a total of 4,333 ED conjunctivitis visits taking place during the period of January 2010 to December 2011 in Calgary, Alberta, Canada. The analysis demonstrated significant associations between exposures to NO_2, $PM_{2.5}$, and O_3 experienced within the 8-day period before the ED visit and the risks of ED visits for conjunctivitis in different population strata. The risks differed by gender, by the latency between exposure and ED visit, and by season (warm vs. cold).

The means and variability (inter-quartile ranges) of pollutants and weather variables in the unique climate and pollution settings in Calgary differed from those examined in other, similar, studies [14, 17, 47]. Overall, Calgary had a warmer average temperature, with less variability than in other Canadian cities [14, 47]. Calgary also had more variability in humidity, with the lowest average humidity—when referring to previous studies of air pollution and ED conjunctivitis visits [14, 18, 47]. NO_2 levels in this study were similar to those levels in previous studies [14, 18, 32, 47]. $PM_{2.5}$ levels were lower than levels in a previous multi-city study in Taiwan [18], but higher than in other, similar studies in Canada [14, 47].

Ozone levels in Calgary warrant additional discussion. The average O_3 was lower than in Taiwan and in Ontario, as seen in the multi-city study and the Canadian studies [18, 47], but higher than in Edmonton, Alberta, Canada [14]. Additionally, there was less variability in the O_3 levels than in the other studies. Higher ground level ozone is typically created on sunny days with warm weather [5, 6]. However, high concentrations of ozone have also been observed during below-freezing temperatures in high-elevation areas similar to Calgary's geography [54].

Thus, levels of O_3 in cold weather months are expected to demonstrate a different pattern of influence on health than the pattern shown in previous studies conducted in sites at lower elevations [18, 32, 47].

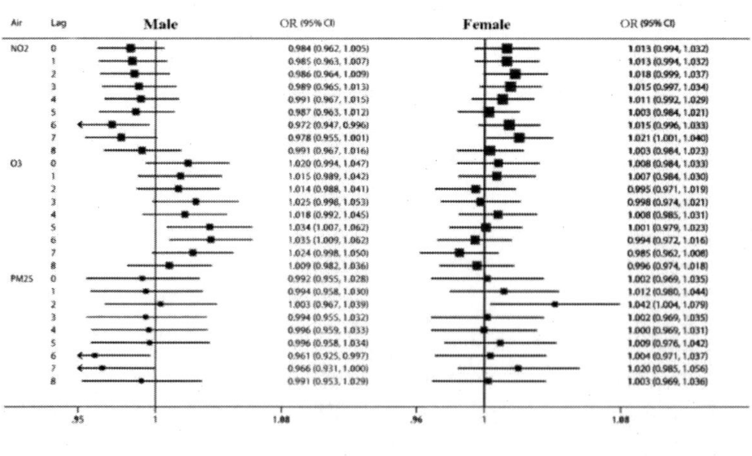

Figure 4. Results for conjunctivitis in Calgary during cold seasons.

In this study, the strongest positive effect of the pollutants on ED conjunctivitis visits was seen in the female population, during warm months, five days after exposure to higher levels of NO_2. Smaller statistically significant effects were still seen up to seven days after exposure. In the cold months, the effects occurred at exactly seven days after the exposure. The latency between exposure and conjunctivitis visit corresponds with the typical incubation period for bacterial conjunctivitis; it is 1-7 days [1]. Exposure to NO_2 may dry and acidify the tear film, a thin protective layer on the eye surface [38, 48, 55, 56]. There are gender differences in the surface acid-base balance of the eye, which may account for the increased susceptibility of females to the biological stressor as the air pollution [57].

The relationship between NO_2 exposure and ED visits for conjunctivitis in the female population is consistent with the findings in previous studies [18, 32, 47]. Applying meta-analysis, pooled estimates from 9 cities across Ontario, Canada, revealed statistically significant positive relationships between increases in ambient NO_2 and ED visits for conjunctivitis 5-8 days after exposure [47]. Other studies have found significant positive relationships, for both genders, between increased levels of NO_2 and visits for conjunctivitis immediately after exposure [18] and up to 2 days after exposure [32]. However, these studies did not examine the latencies longer than 3 ([32]) and 5 days ([18]).

NO_2 levels were associated with conjunctivitis-related male ED visits in an unexpected direction. Exposure to higher levels of NO_2 decreased the risk of ED conjunctivitis visits 4 days after exposure in warm months and six days after exposure in cold months. It is noteworthy that the relationship between pollutant levels and ED visits for conjunctivitis may not be linear. Most of the less acute eye irritations are treated at home with over-the-counter and self-care regimens [58]. It is plausible that low-level irritations, if any, decrease the risk for ED visits while self-care interventions are utilized, while sub-clinically resolving infections increases a later risk for infection [58].

The relationship between NO_2 and ED visits for conjunctivitis among males found in this study is not consistent with findings in previous studies [18, 32, 47]. This study was based on a smaller sample (less than 5,000 visits) than previous studies (>30,000 visits) [18, 32, 47]. The specific climate in Calgary, or the weaker statistical power of the sample may explain the inconsistency. In this study, a relationship between increased concentrations of O_3 and ED visits for conjunctivitis during warm months has not been found. However, there was a statistically significant positive relationship, found for the male population and cold weather, when examining the visits occurring 5 or 6 days after exposure. O_3 is thought to directly impact the homeostasis of protective mucus membranes by causing oxidative stress, directly damaging cells and inducting tissue inflammation [21-29]. Previous studies demonstrated various relationships between increased O_3 concentrations and ED visits for conjunctivitis: for both genders and for shorter lags (0-1 days) [18, 32]; only for males, at lags 0-3 and 7 [47]; for both genders, but not for the male sample, at lags 5 and 7. Clarification of inconsistencies in these results, particularly in the timing of ED visit after the exposure, may indicate at the need for more study on the interactions between conjunctivitis morbidity and environmental conditions. It is plausible that the elevation, and interactions with cold-weather ozone formation, impacted the observed relationships.

Increased concentrations of $PM_{2.5}$ were associated with an increase in counts of ED visits for conjunctivitis, for males, six days after exposure, in warm weather months. For females, higher count of the visits two days after exposure, in cold weather months, was noticed. There was also an association of the increased concentrations of $PM_{2.5}$ with decreased counts of ED visits for conjunctivitis, for males, six days after exposure, in cold weather months. Particulate matter may carry infectious or allergic agents directly into the eye surface [59] and is correlated with increased production of the aqueous (or watery) part of the tear film [60, 61], oxidative stress and inflammation [62], and an increase in debris at the eyelid margins [60].

Typical environmental measures of particulate matter incidence do not reveal the composition of the particulates. They may be chemical pollutants, organic irritants, or inorganic dust. Previous studies have also reported associations between $PM_{2.5}$ occurrences and ED visits for conjunctivitis: for males 5 days after exposures [47] and for females 6-7 days after exposure [47]. Also it has been stated that there was no relationship [18]. No studies reported a decreased risk for ED conjunctivitis (we have found such relation in the male population, during cold weather). Specific particulate matters may trigger unpredictable health responses; further studies are needed to elucidate the role of the confounders as a particular composition of PM.

Non-significant or conflicting results reported in this study may reflect our inability to accurately describe conjunctivitis etiology. This study includes the ED visits for several types of conjunctivitis: non-specific, allergic, and infectious. In the ED clinical care, differentiating the types of conjunctivitis is most often based on physical exam and on the history of a cluster of, frequently, non-specific symptoms [1]. Once the rare and most damaging etiologies are ruled out, a broad range of treatment approaches, supported by the current clinical evidence, are still possible.

Depending on the severity and duration of symptoms, the clinician is justified in most cases in either prescribing immediate treatment, or in no treatment with the expectation the conjunctivitis to self-resolve, or in watchful waiting for a specified follow-up period [1]. Thus, specifying the type of conjunctivitis is not always relevant to ED clinical treatment. However, the different causes (allergic, viral, and bacterial) of conjunctivitis are likely to have very different correlations with air pollutants.

This study has several limitations, common to ecologically-based research, which should be considered and addressed in future research. The results demonstrate correlation, not causation, among the variables. However, testing at different lags adds evidence of the temporal nature of exposure versus health outcome. This study likely underestimated the impact of air pollution on conjunctivitis, since most eye irritation is treated through self-care methods; the count of ED visit is not a fully reliable measure of the morbidity of conjunctivitis. Centralized air monitoring stations measured average population exposure and not personal exposure for the individual who presented to the ED with conjunctivitis. However, personal monitors for a city-wide study are not currently feasible. Each lag tested is a separate statistical test on the same data, increasing the risk for Type I statistical errors.

Finally, using ICD-10 codes from billing claims are subject to misclassification of the true etiology for conjunctivitis.

In conclusion, our study supports the claims that there are associations between air pollutant concentrations and ED visits for conjunctivitis. We differentiated the relationship between exposure and outcome by gender, season, and latency period.

The results concerning exposure to NO_2 and ED visit for conjunctivitis among females are consistent with the results of previous studies. However, several key inconsistencies in the findings create the need for additional research to determine the cause-and-effect relationship between the exposure to air pollutants and the etiology of bacterial conjunctivitis.

Acknowledgments

The authors thank Dr. Mieczysław Szyszkowicz for helpful discussion, suggestions, and advice in the methodology.

The authors acknowledge Patricia H. Garman Behavioral Health Nursing Endowment Fund at the University at Buffalo’s School of Nursing and

Environment Canada for providing the air pollution data from the National Air Pollution Surveillance (NAPS) network that was used in this study.

REFERENCES

[1] Azari, A. A., Barney, N. P. Conjunctivitis: a systematic review of diagnosis and treatment. *JAMA Ophthalmol*. 2013;310:1721-1730.

[2] Rozanova, E., Heilig, P., Godnic-Cvar, J. The eye--a neglected organ in environmental and occupational medicine: an overview of known environmental and occupational non-traumatic effects on the eyes. *Arh. Hig. Rada. Toksikol*. 2009;60:205-215.

[3] Stokols, D. Translating social ecological theory into guidelines for community health promotion. *Am. J. Health Promot*. 1996;10:282–298. doi: 10.4278/0890-1171-10.4.282.

[4] McLeroy, K. R., Bibeau, D., Steckler, A., Glanz, K. An ecological perspective on health promotion programs. *Health Educ. Quart*. 1988;15 (4):351–377. doi: 10.1177/109019818801500401.

[5] Environment Canada. *Canadian Environmental Protection Act*, 1999. http://www.ec.gc.ca/lcpe-cepa/default.asp?lang=Enandn=CC0DE5E2-1andtoc=hide. Accessed April 1, 2014.

[6] US Environmental Protection Agency. *The plain English guide to the clean air act*. 2007: Publication # EPA-456/k-07-001.

[7] US Environmental Protection Agency. *Technology Transfer Network. National Ambient Air Quality Standard*. http://www.epa.gov/ttn/naaqs/. Accessed November 21, 2013.

[8] Villeneuve, P. J., Chen, L., Rowe, B. H., Coates, F. Outdoor air pollution and emergency department visits for asthma among children and adults: a case-crossover study in northern Alberta, Canada. *Environ. Health*. 2007;6:40.

[9] Stieb, D. M., Szyszkowicz, M., Rowe, B. H., Leech, J. A. Air pollution and emergency department visits for cardiac and respiratory conditions: a multi-city time-series analysis. *Environ. Health*. 2009;8:25.

[10] Wong, T. W., Lau, T. S., Yu, T. S., Neller, A., Wong, S. L., Tam, W., et al. Air pollution and hospital admissions for respiratory and cardiovascular diseases in Hong Kong. *Occup. Environ. Med*. 1999;56: 679–683.

[11] Kaplan, G. G., Dixon, E., Panaccione, R., Fong, A., Chen, L., Szyszkowicz, M., et al. Effect of ambient air pollution on the incidence of appendicitis. *CMAJ*. 2009;181:591–597.

[12] Szyszkowicz, M., Kaplan, G. G., Grafstein, E., Rowe, B. H. Emergency department visits for migraine and headache: a multi-city study. *Int. J. Occup. Med. Environ. Health*. 2009;22:235–242.

[13] Larrieu, S., Lefranc, A., Gault, G., Chatignoux, E., Couvy, F., Jouves, B. Are the short-term effects of air pollution restricted to cardiorespiratory diseases? *Am. J. Epidemiol*. 2009; 169:1201-8.

[14] Szyszkowicz, M., Porada, E., Searles, G., Rowe, B. H. Ambient ozone and emergency department visits for skin conditions. *Air Qual. Atmos. Health*. 2012;5:303-309.

[15] Xu, F., Yan, S., Wu, M., Li, F., Xu, X., Song, W., et al. Ambient ozone pollution as a risk factor for skin disorders. *Br. J. Dermatol*. 2011;165: 224-5.

[16] Szyszkowicz, M., Porada, E., Kaplan, G. G., Rowe, B. H. Ambient ozone and emergency department visits for cellulitis. *Int. J. Environ. Res. Public Health*. 2010;7(11):4078-88.

[17] Szyszkowicz, M., Porada, E., Grafstein, E., Rowe, B. H. Ambient ozone as a risk factor for ED visits for cellulitis. *Environment and Pollution*. 2012;1:2:105-111.

[18] Chang, C. J., Yang, H. H., Chang, C. A., Tsai, H. Y. Relationship between Air Pollution and Outpatient Visits for Nonspecific Conjunctivitis. *Invest. Ophthal. and Vis. Sci*. 2012; 53: 429–433.

[19] US Environmental Protection Agency. *Air quality index: a guide to air quality and your health*. http://www.epa.gov/airnow/aqi_brochure_08-09.pdf. Published August, 2009. Accessed November 21, 2013.

[20] US Environmental Protection Agency. *AIR Trends 1995 Summary, Particulate Matter (PM-10)*. http://www.epa.gov/airtrends/aqtrnd95/pm10.html. Accessed November 13, 2013.

[21] Valacchi, G., Fortino, V., Bocci, V. The dual action of ozone on the skin. *Br. J. Dermatol*. 2005;153: 1096–1100.

[22] Fridovich, I. The biology of oxygen radicals. *Science*. 1978;201:875–880.

[23] Aris, R. M., Christian, D., Hearne, P. Q., Kerr, K., Finkbeiner, W. E., Balmes, J. R. Ozone-induced airway inflammation in human subjects as determined by airway lavage and biopsy. *Am. Rev. Respir. Dis*. 1993; 148:1363–1372.

[24] Pryor, W. A. Ozone in all its reactive splendor. *J. Lab. Clin. Med.* 1993; 122:483–486.

[25] Camhi, S. L., Lee, P., Choi, A. M. The oxidative stress response. *New Hor.* 1995;3:170–182.

[26] Devlin, R. B., Raub, J. A., Folinsbee, L. J. Health effects of ozone. *Sci. Med.* 1997;8–17.

[27] Devlin, R. B., McDonnell, W. F., Mann, R., Becker, S., House, D. E., Schreinemachers, D., et al. Exposure of human to ambient levels of ozone for 6.6 hours causes cellular and biochemical changes in the lung. *Am. J. Respir. Cell Mol. Biol.* 1991;4:72–81.

[28] Devlin, R. B., McKinnon, K. R., Noah, T., Becker, S., Koren, H. S. Ozone-induced release of cytokines and fibronectin by alveolar macrophages and airway epithelial cells. *Am. J. Physiol.* 1994;266: L612–L619.

[29] Morrison, D., Rahman, I., Macnee, W. Permeability, inflammation and oxidant status in airspace epithelium exposed to ozone. *Respir. Med.* 2006;100:2227–2234.

[30] Burnett, R. T., Smith-Doiron, M., Stieb, D., Raizenne, M. E., Brook, J. R., Dales, R. E., et al. Association between ozone and hospitalization for acute respiratory diseases in children less than 2 years of age. *Am. J. Epidemiol.* 2001;153:444–452.

[31] Chang, C. J., Yang, H. H., Chang, C. A., Tsai, H. Y. Volatile Organic Compounds and Nonspecific Conjunctivitis: A Population-Based Study. *Aerosol Air Qual. Res.* 2013;13:237-242.

[32] Bourcier, T., Viboud, C., Cohen, J. C., Thomas, F., Bury, T., Cadiot, L., et al. Effects of air pollution and climatic conditions on the frequency of ophthalmological emergency examinations. *Br. J. Ophthalmol.* 2003; 87: 809-811.

[33] Waheed, M. A., Basu, P. K. The effect of air pollutants on the eye. I. The effect of an organic extract on the conjunctival goblet cells. *Can. J. Ophthalmol.* 1970;5:226-30.

[34] Artridge, R. A., Stebbings, J. H. Jr, Elsea, W. R., Winkelstein, W. Jr. Outbreak of acute eye irritation associated with air pollution. *Public Health Rep.* 1966;81:153-8.

[35] Altshuller, A. P. Eye irritation as an effect of photochemical air pollution. *J. Air Pollut. Control Assoc.* 1977;27:1125-6.

[36] Basu, P. K. Air pollution and the eye. *Surv. Ophthalmol.* 1972;17:78-93.

[37] Lemp, M. A. Report of the National Eye Institute/Industry Workshop on clinical trials in dry eyes. *CLAO J.* 1995;21:221-32.

[38] Versura, P., Profazio, V., Cellini, M., Torreggiani, A., Caramazza, R. Eye discomfort and air pollution. *Ophthalmologica*. 1999;213:103-9.

[39] Klopfer, J. Effects of environmental air pollution on the eye. *J. Am. Optom. Assoc.* 1989;60:773-8.

[40] Andrés, S., Garcia, M. L., Espina, M., Valero, J., Valls, O. Tear pH, air pollution, and contact lenses. *Am. J. Optom. Physiol. Opt*. 1988;65:627-31.

[41] Wolkoff, P., Skov, P., Franck, C., Petersen, L. N. Eye irritation and environmental factors in the office environment-hypotheses, causes and a physiological model. *Scand. J. Work Environ. Health*. 2003;29:411-30.

[42] Schneider, T., Bohgard, M. Airborne particle deposition onto the ocular surface. *Indoor Air*. 2005;15:215-19.

[43] Kiesswetter, E., van Thriel, C., Schaeper, M., Blaszkewicz, M., Seeber, A. Eye blinks as indicator for sensory irritation during constant and peak exposures to 2-ethylhexanol. *Environ. Toxicol. Pharmacol.* 2005;19: 531-41.

[44] Novaes, P., do Nascimento Saldiva, P. H., Kara-José, N., Macchione, M., Matsuda, M., Racca, L., et al. Ambient levels of air pollution induce goblet-cell hyperplasia in human conjunctival epithelium. *Environ. Health Perspect.* 2007;115:1753-6.

[45] Wittenborn, J., Zhang, X., Feagan, C., Crouse, W., Shrestha, S., Kemper, A., et al. The economic burden of vision loss and eye disorders among the United States population younger than 40 years. *Ophthalmology*. 2013;120:1728-1735.

[46] Bielory, L., Meltzer, E. O., Nichols, K. K., Melton, R., Thomas, R. K., Bartlett, J. D. An algorithm for the management of allergic conjunctivitis. *Allergy Asthma Proc*. 2013;34:408-420.

[47] Szyszkowicz, M., Kousha, T., Castner, J. *Air pollution and emergency department visits for conjunctivitis: A case crossover study*. Population studies division, Health Canada.

[48] Calgary Region Airshed Zone (CRAZ), *Annual report 2009*. http://www.craz.ca/assets/fileManager/Reports/2009%20CRAZ%20Annual%20Report.pdf.

[49] Canadian Institute for Health Information. [Internet]. Ottawa: 2013 [cited 2014, Mar. 7]. Available from: www.cihi.ca.

[50] Environment Canada. [Internet]. Gatineau: 2013 [cited 2014, Mar. 7]. Available from: http://www.ec.gc.ca/rnspa-naps/.

[51] Maclure, M. The case-crossover design: a method for studying transient effects on the risk of acute events. *Am. J. Epidemiol.* 1991;133(2):144-153.

[52] Janes, H., Sheppard, L., Lumley, T. Case-crossover analyses of air pollution exposure data. Referent selection strategies and their implications for bias. *Epidemiology*. 2005;16(6): 717-726.

[53] Bateson, T. F., Schwartz, J. Control for seasonal variation and time trend in case-crossover studies of acute effects of environmental exposures. *Epidemiology* 1999;10:539–44.

[54] US Environmental Protection Agency. *What is ozone?* http://www.epa.gov/groundlevelozone/designations/faq.htm. Accessed April 1, 2014.

[55] Saxena, R., Srivastava, S., Trivedi, D., Anand, E., Joshi, S., Gupta, S. K. Impact of environmental pollution on the eye. *Acta Ophthalmol.* Suppl. 2003;81:491-494.

[56] Gupta, S. K., Gupta, V., Joshi, S., Tandon, R. Subclinically dry eyes in urban Delhi: An impact of air pollution? *Ophthalmologica*. 2002; 216: 368-71.

[57] Coles, W. H., Jaros, P. A. Dynamics of ocular surface ph. *Br. J. Ophthalmol.* 1984;68:549-552.

[58] Bielory, L., Syed, B. A. Pharmacoeconomics of anterior ocular inflammatory disease. *Curr. Opin. Allergy Clin. Immunol.* 2013;13:537-542.

[59] Sandstrom, T., Forsberg, B. Desert dust: an unrecognized source of dangerous air pollution? *Epidemiology*. 2008;19;808-9.

[60] Malerbi, F. K., Martins, L. C., Saldiva, P. H., Braga, A. L. Ambient levels of air pollution induce clinical worsening of blepharitis. *Environ. Res. J.* 2012;112:199-203.

[61] Torricelli, A. A., Novaes, P., Matsuda, M., Braga, A., Saldiva, P. H., Alves, M. R., et al. Correlation between signs and symptoms of ocular surface dysfunction and tear osmolarity with ambient levels of air pollution in a large metropolitan area. *Cornea*. 2013;32:e11-e15.

[62] Liu, H., Begley, C., Chen, M., Bradley, A., Bonanno, J., McNamara, N. A link between tear instability and hyperosmolarity in dry eye. *Invest. Ophthalmol. Vis. Sci*. 2009;50:3671-3679.

[63] Hori, Y., Maeda, N., Sakamoto, M., Koh, S., Inoue, T., Tano, Y. Bacteriologic profile of the conjunctiva in patients with dry eye. *Am. J. Ophthalmol.* 2008;146:729-734.

In: Conjunctivitis
Editor: Elias H. Bazile
ISBN: 978-1-63321-621-1

Chapter 4

Bacterial Conjunctivitis in Childhood: Etiology, Clinical Manifestations, Diagnosis and Management

Alexander K. C. Leung[1*], Kam Lun Hon[2] and Alex H. C. Wong[3]

[1]MBBS, FRCPC, FRCP(UK & Irel), FRCPCH, FAAP, Clinical Professor, Department of Pediatrics, University of Calgary, Pediatric Consultant, Alberta Children's Hospital, Calgary, Alberta, Canada

[2]MD, FAAP, Professor, Department of Paediatrics, Chinese University of Hong Kong Hong Kong, SAR

[3]MD, CCFP, Clinical Assistant Professor, Department of Family Medicine, University of Calgary, Calgary, Alberta, Canada

Abstract

Bacterial conjunctivitis is common in childhood and accounts for 1 to 2% of primary care encounters. In the neonatal period, the most common causative organism is *Staphylococcus aureus* followed by

* Address correspondence to: Dr. Alexander K.C. Leung, #200, 233 – 16th Avenue NW, Calgary, Alberta, Canada T2M 0H5, Telefax: (403) 230-3322, e-mail: aleung@ucalgary.ca.

Chlamydia trachomatis. Other organisms include *Haemophilus influenzae*, *Streptococcus pneumoniae*, and *Neisseria gonorrhoeae*. In children, bacterial conjunctivitis is most often caused by *H. influenzae*, *S. pneumoniae*, and *Moraxella catarrhalis.* Clinically, bacterial conjunctivitis is characterized by purulent ocular discharge, eye crusting or sticky eyes on awakening, foreign body sensation, and conjunctival injection. In more severe cases, chemosis and lid edema may also occur. The involvement is usually unilateral at first but rapidly spreads to the contralateral eye. The diagnosis is mainly clinically. Cultures along with Gram or Giemsa stains should be considered in neonatal conjunctivitis, conjunctivitis presenting with severe purulent discharge, suspected venereal infections, immunodeficiency, recurrent cases, or cases that fail to respond to therapy. While it is beyond doubt that conjunctivitis caused by *C. trachomatis* or *N. gonorrhoeae* needs to be treated, some authors suggest a watchful observation approach to other bacterial causes of conjunctivitis as most other cases of bacterial conjunctivitis are self-limited. A recent Cochrane review, however, suggests that the use of antibiotic eye drops is associated with modestly improved rates of clinical and microbiological remission in comparison to the use of placebo. The present consensus supports prompt use of topical antibiotics as they shorten the course of the disease, reduce the discomfort associated with the infection, reduce the risk of ocular damage, prevent person-to-person transmission, and reduce rate of re-infection.

Keywords: Conjunctivitis, childhood, bacteria, ocular discharge, conjunctival injection, topical antibiotics

INTRODUCTION

Bacterial conjunctivitis is a common cause for consultation in pediatric practices and is a significant healthcare concern. The condition is characterized by purulent ocular discharge, matting of the eyelids on awakening, burning, stinging or foreign body sensation, and conjunctival injection.

Bacterial conjunctivitis has to be differentiated from other causes of conjunctivitis such as viral conjunctivitis and allergic conjunctivitis. As treatment is specific for each etiology, a correct diagnosis is important so that appropriate treatment can be instituted.

A review of the topic is therefore in order and is the purpose of the present chapter.

EPIDEMIOLOGY

In western world, the prevalence of acute infective conjunctivitis is estimated to be 13 to 15 cases per 1000 persons per year [1]. Bacterial conjunctivitis is a common cause of conjunctivitis and accounts for up to 50% of all cases of acute infective conjunctivitis in adults and 70 to 80% of all cases in children [2, 3]. The condition accounts for 1 to 2% of primary care encounters [3, 4]. The 2005 National Medical Survey in the United States estimated the incidence of bacterial conjunctivitis at 1.35% [5]. Bacterial conjunctivitis is observed more frequently in winter and spring [6-8].

Bacterial conjunctivitis is highly contagious [9]. Common routes of transmission include contaminated fingers, contaminated fomites, and oculogenital spread [6, 10]. Predisposing factors include poor personal hygiene, day-care or school attendance, compromised tear production, blocked nasolacrimal duct, trauma, wearing of contact lens, pre-existing ocular surface disease, and immunodeficiency [9].

ETIOLOGY

The bacteria causing neonatal conjunctivitis are different from those causing conjunctivitis in older children because neonates often acquire the bacteria during passage through the birth canal or in the hospital environment [3]. In the neonatal period, the most common causative organism is *Staphylococcus aureus* followed by *Chlamydia trachomatis*. In one study, *S. aureus* accounted for 65% of all cases of neonatal conjunctivitis [11]. Approximately one-third of neonates born vaginally to mothers with untreated *C. trachomatis* infection develop conjunctivitis [12, 13]. Other organisms include *Staphylococcus epidermidis*, *Haemophilus influenzae*, *Streptococcus pneumoniae*, *Moraxella catarrhalis*, and *Neisseria gonorrhoeae* [13]. Gonococcal conjunctivitis is rarely seen nowadays due to the routine instillation of ocular prophylaxis with erythromycin, silver nitrate or povidone-iodine at birth.

In children, bacterial conjunctivitis is most often caused by *H. influenzae* (nontypeable *H. influenzae* being the most common organism), followed by *S. pneumoniae*, and *M. catarrhalis* [14-17]. Other less common bacterial organisms include *S. aureus*, coagulase negative staphylococci, *Escherichia coli*, *Corynebacterium* species, and *Pseudomonas aeruginosa* [4, 13, 18].

P. aeruginosa is the most common causative organism in individuals who wear contact lens [19]. In adolescents, Staphylococci predominate [20]. *N. gonorrhoeae* and *C. trachomatis* may cause conjunctivitis in sexually active individuals [1, 20].

Clinical Manifestations

In the majority of cases, the incubation period is 1 to 7 days [10]. In childhood, bacterial conjunctivitis is characterized by purulent ocular discharge, eye crusting or sticky or glued eyes on awakening, burning, stinging or foreign body sensation, and, conjunctival injection [16, 21]. Because of the conjunctival injection, the condition is commonly referred to as "red eye" or "pink eye" by the lay public. The discharge is often yellow or green in color. In more severe cases, chemosis and lid edema may also occur. The involvement is usually unilateral at first but spreads rapidly to the contralateral eye [3, 21]. Pruritus is either mild or absent.

Age 6 years or older, absence of sticky or glued eyes on awakening, no or watery ocular discharge, and presentation from April through November are variables that may help to identify children at low risk for bacterial conjunctivitis [22]. A history of recent conjunctivitis also argues against bacterial conjunctivitis [15]. In addition, ocular pain, photophobia, hazy cornea, restriction of ocular movement, impaired visual acuity, ciliary flush, and proptosis are not features of bacterial conjunctivitis and other causes should be considered [23].

In children, acute bacterial conjunctivitis is sometimes associated with otitis media (conjunctivitis-otitis syndrome) [3,24]. This is most often caused by nontypeable *H. influenzae* [17]. Sinusitis and rhinitis can accompany conjunctivitis caused by pneumococci [17].

For neonatal ophthalmia, gonococcal ophthalmia typically occurs around 2 to 5 days after birth [12]. The disease is rapidly progressive with copious, thick, yellow-green, purulent ocular discharge, eyelid swelling, chemosis, pseudomembrane formation, preauricular lymphadenopathy, and possible corneal involvement [13]. Chamydial ophthalmia, on the other hand, usually occurs 5 to 14 days after delivery or earlier if there is premature rupture of amniotic membranes [12,13]. The disease may manifest as mild conjunctival injection with scant mucoid discharge to severe mucopurulent conjunctivitis with chemosis and pseudomembrane formation [12]. Conjunctival hyperemia, mucopurulent ocular discharge, and lymphoid follicle formation are hallmarks of chamydial conjunctivitis [6]. Vaginal delivery, premature rupture of amniotic membranes, prolonged labor, and history of midwife interference increase the risk for neonatal conjunctivitis [25]. On the other hand, breast milk has a protective effect [26].

Laboratory Investigations

Routine eye swabs are uncomfortable and impractical (on grounds of delay and cost) in most settings and are not commonly performed. Cultures along with Gram or Giemsa stains should be considered in neonatal conjunctivitis, conjunctivitis presenting with severe purulent discharge, suspected venereal infections, immunodeficiency, outbreaks, recurrent cases, or in cases that fail to respond to therapy [6, 12, 14, 27].

Diagnosis and Differential Diagnosis

The diagnosis is mainly clinical. The differential diagnosis include viral conjunctivitis, seasonal and perennial allergic conjunctivitis, vernal keratoconjunctivitis, atopic keratoconjunctivitis, giant papillary conjunctivitis, subconjunctival hemorrhage, keratitis, scleritis, uveitis, glaucoma, corneal abrasion, and Kawasaki disease.

Viral conjunctivitis is usually bilateral in onset and frequently associated an upper respiratory infection (e.g. runny nose, cough) [21]. Serous ophthalmic discharge, pharyngeal erythema, fever, preauricular lymphadenopathy suggest viral conjunctivitis. It should be noted that any viral conjunctivitis may be complicated by bacterial conjunctivitis [23].

Seasonal and perennial allergic conjunctivitis are IgE-mediated, immediate hypersensitivity conditions characterized by ocular pruritus, epiphora (tearing), and hyperemia [28]. Ocular/peri-ocular pruritus is pathognomonic, without which the ocular condition is unlikely to be an ocular allergy [29]. Other symptoms may include conjunctival burning, stinging, epiphora, eyelid swelling, and photophobia. Some patients report gritty, foreign body sensations in the eyes. On examination, the conjunctiva may demonstrate hyperemia (injection) and chemosis [29]. Peri-orbital edema is a sign of acute ocular allergy. Lid edema, mucous discharge, and papillary hypertrophy along the tarsal conjunctival surface may sometimes occur. Dark circles under the eyes, as a result of venous congestion, can sometimes be seen [30,31]. Features of other allergic or atopic co-morbidities such as allergic rhinitis, atopic dermatitis, and asthma may coexist [30-32].

Vernal (springtime) keratoconjunctivitis is a chronic bilateral ocular inflammatory process mediated mainly by the Th2-lymphocyte. The tears of affected patients have high levels of IgE and mast cell mediators such as histamine. It generally affects children and young adolescents and is more common in males and in the warm months (hence the term "vernal"). The disease is characterized by intense ocular itching, redness, swelling, foreign body sensation, photophobia, mucus discharge, and tearing [33]. Physical examination often shows giant papillae (usually a few mm in diameter) on the upper tarsal conjunctiva giving rise to a cobblestone appearance, and they can be seen easily by “flipping” the upper eyelid. There may be a tenacious white fibrinous discharge between the giant papillae, yellow-white dots on the conjunctiva/limbus, Dennie’s line, and corneal ulcers [28]. Affected patients may have impaired vision. The condition usually resolves by 20 years of age.

Atopic keratoconjunctivitis is an ocular manifestation of atopic dermatitis [22]. The condition is characterized by intense ocular itching, burning, and tearing. Physical examination may show lid eczema, conjunctival injection, chemosis, and papillary hypertrophy on the lower tarsal conjunctiva. Atopic keratoconjunctivitis can persist through life-time.

Giant papillary conjunctivitis is a chronic immune response to long-term exposure to inert substances (e.g. contact lenses, limbal sutures, ocular prostheses) rather than allergens in the eyes. The condition is characterized by papillary hypertrophy of the superior tarsal conjunctiva. There is no significant corneal involvement. Affected patients may present with mucoid eye discharge, itchy foreign body sensation in the eyes, and conjunctival hyperemia.

Subconjunctival hemorrhage is characterized by the acute appearance of a sharply circumscribed ocular redness due to bleeding underneath the conjunctiva in the absence of pain, ocular discharge, inflammation in contagious areas, and visual impairment [34]. The cause is often idiopathic and spontaneous, but it may be secondary to severe coughing, straining, hypertension, and bleeding diathesis.

Characteristic features of keratitis include ocular pain, photophobia, diminished vision, foreign body sensation, and corneal opacity/white spot. Punctate lesions may be seen with fluorescein staining, especially with slit lamp examination [23]. The condition is often secondary to trauma or wearing contact lens [35].

Scleritis is characterized by severe ocular pain radiating to peiorbital area, ocular pain increases with eye movement, ocular tenderness, diminished vision, photophobia, conjunctival injection with dilated vessels, and scleral edema [14, 35]. The condition is often associated with systemic diseases such as rheumatoid arthritis and inflammatory bowel disease [14, 35].

Uveitis is characterized by acute onset of ocular pain radiating into the brow/temple, watery red eyes, photophobia, blurred vision, ocular tenderness, ciliary injection around the limbus, meiotic and irregular pupil, and decreased intraocular pressure [35, 36]. The condition is the most frequent extra-articular feature in seronegative arthritis and there is a strong association with HLA-B27 [36]. Posterior uveitis is more frequently diagnosed in Behcet disease [36].

Narrow-angle glaucoma can present with severe ocular pain, systemic symptoms (such as headache, nausea, vomiting), color haloes around lights, a sluggish or fixed papillary response, visual impairment, and cloudy cornea [35]. Because of the increased intraocular pressure, the eyeball is firm and tender to palpation.

Corneal abrasion is characterized by severe ocular pain, tearing, photophobia, and decreased vision. The abrasion can be detected by instilling fluorescein dye and inspecting the cornea using a blue-filtered light [28].

Kawasaki disease is an acute multisystem vasculitic syndrome of unknown etiology that predominantly affects coronary arteries and occurs mostly in children younger than 5 years of age. Kawasaki disease is characterized by fever that last for at least five days, conjunctival injection, oral mucosal changes, swelling and edema of the hands and feet with stretched and shiny skin, a sharp demarcation at the ankles and wrists with an abrupt change to normal skin, desquamation of the fingers and toes, Beau lines at the nail base, polymorphous rash, and cervical lymphadenopathy [37].

COMPLICATIONS

Bacterial conjunctivitis has a significant economic and social impact resulting from disruption of the patient's normal activities such as reading and computer use and absenteeism from school or from work [38]. It also has an adverse effect on the patient's quality of life. Otitis media develops in approximately 25% of children with *H. influenzae* conjunctivitis [15, 24]. Other complications include orbital cellulitis and keratitis (especially in contact lens wearers) [1, 18]. Untreated gonococcal ophthalmia neonatorum may cause corneal ulceration/perforation, endophthalmitis, and panophthalmitis [1, 15, 18]. Untreated chlamydial conjunctivitis may lead to corneal and conjunctival scarring [12].

PROGNOSIS

Mild forms of bacterial conjunctivitis is usually self-limiting. Even without treatment, the condition usually resolves in approximately 7 days [14, 39]. Severe complications are rare [14, 39]. A Cochrane systematic review showed that clinical remission occurs within 2 to 5 days in 65% (95% confidence interval: 59% to 70%) of microbiologically confirmed cases treated with placebo [40]. The use of topical antibiotic increases the likelihood of early clinical remission and microbiological remission [41].

PREVENTION

At birth, prophylactic topical erythromycin ointment is routinely given to all newborns to prevent gonococcal conjunctivitis and chlamydial conjunctivitis [42, 43].

Compared to topical silver nitrate, topical erythromycin ointment has a low risk for chemical conjunctivitis [43]. Compared to other topical antibiotics, topical povidone-iodine is less acceptable to parents because of tinting of the sclera.

Prophylactic topical antibiotic, however, will not totally eradicate conjunctivitis caused by *C. trachomatis* [42]. Presumably, this is due to its lack of deeper penetration into the conjunctival tissue [42]. Nevertheless, the risk of developing chlamydial conjunctivitis is reduced dramatically if erythromycin ointment is applied within one hour of delivery [13]. On the other hand, gonococcal ophthalmia neonatorum can occur in up to 10% of infants exposed to gonorrheal exudate in the birth canal despite topical prophylaxis [15].

Therefore, infants born to mothers with gonorrhea should receive a single dose of parenteral ceftriaxone for prophylaxis [13]. The recommended dose is 125 mg for term infants and 25 to 50 mg/kg (not to exceed 125 mg) for preterm and low-birth weight infants [13].

MANAGEMENT

The eye discharge should be cleaned by wiping from the bridge of the nose to the outer eye, using a fresh piece of cotton wool or gauze for each wipe [44]. Eye rubbing should be discouraged. Hand washing and avoiding the sharing of towels or personal items should be emphasized. Patient wearing contact lens should be advised not to wear contact lens until the infection has subsided.

While it is beyond doubt that conjunctivitis caused by *C. trachomatis* or *N. gonorrhoeae* needs to be treated, some authors suggest a benign neglect approach to other bacterial causes of conjunctivitis as most other cases of bacterial conjunctivitis are self-limited. A recent Cochrane meta-analysis of six double-blind, randomized controlled trials on patients with acute bacterial conjunctivitis (n = 1057), however, suggests that the use of antibiotic eye drops is associated with modestly improved rates of clinical remission (risk ratio: 1.36; 95% confidence interval: 1.15 to 1.61) and microbiological remission (risk ratio: 1.55; 95% confidence interval: 1.37 to 1.76) in comparison to the use of placebo (n = 1059) [41]. The present consensus supports prompt use of topical antibiotics as they shorten the course of the disease, reduce the discomfort associated with the infection, accelerate return to normal activities, reduce the risk of complications, enhance eradication of the causative organisms, prevent person-to-person transmission, and reduce rate of re-infection [18]. Many health departments in the United States mandate that students with conjunctivitis, regardless of the underlying cause, to be treated with topical antibiotic eye drops before they are allowed to return to school [45].

The antibiotics chosen should be broad-spectrum and effective against a variety of pathogens because the exact microbial is not usually known [3]. In addition, the agents should have a rapid bactericidal activity, achieve a high concentration in the eye, have a long residual time at the infection site, are well tolerated, and have a favorable safety profile [18, 19]. In this regard, topical chloramphenicol is best avoided because of the risk of systemic complications, though rare, from the absorption of the medication into the general circulation through the conjunctival mucosa. Aplastic anemia, grey baby syndrome, and acute hepatitis have been reported following the topical administration of chloramphenicol eye drops [10, 46, 47]. Ophthalmic suspensions are often used instead of ophthalmic ointments. The latter are not usually preferred due to difficulty with vision after its application and difficulty manipulating the agents [3]. Other factors that should be taken into considerations in the choice of topical antibiotics are cost-effectiveness, local availability, local bacterial resistance data, patient allergy, patient compliance as well as patient preference as some eye drops may cause too much eye stinging pain or irritation.

The classes of topical ophthalmic antimicrobial agents available for the treatment of acute bacterial conjunctivitis include polymyxin B combinations (polymyxin B/neomycin/gramicidin, polymyxin B/bacitracin, polymyxin B/ trimethoprim, neomycin/trimethoprim/bacitracin), macrolides (erythromycin, azithromycin), aminoglycosides (tobramycin, gentamycin, neomycin), and fluoroquinolones (ciprofloxacin, ofloxacin, norfloxacin, gatifloxacin, moxifloxacin, besifloxcin) [1, 20, 48]. Polymyxin B is effective against only gram-positive organisms and is therefore administered in combination with other antibiotics with complementary modes of action to provide a broader spectrum of coverage [9]. The polymyxin B combinations penetrate tissue poorly and are not reliably bactericidal [18]. Macrolides inhibit protein synthesis but do not affect nucleic acid synthesis and are therefore bacteriostatic rather than bactericidal. In addition, erythromycin has good gram-positive coverage with the exception of enterococci but poor activity against *H. influenzae* and *Staphylococcus* species [2, 48]. Although azithromycin is a newer macrolide, it shows little activity against methicillin-resistant *S. aureus* (MRSA) [48]. Nevertheless, it has been shown that azithromycin 1.5% ophthalmic solution is not inferior to tobramycin 0.3% ophthalmic solution in the treatment of purulent bacterial conjunctivitis [49, 50]. Because of its sustained and high intracellular penetration and tissue concentration as well as prolonged bioavailability, the recommended dosage of azithromycin 1.5% ophthalmic solution is one drop in the affected eye twice a day for 3 days [50]. The less frequent dosage schedule and the short treatment course would increase patient compliance and improve the quality of life [49]. The aminoglycosides are bactericidal and effective against gram-negative bacteria, particularly *P. aeruginosa* (with the exception of neomycin), but provide incomplete coverage against gram-positive bacteria [9, 18]. In addition, their potential to cause reactive keratoconjunctivitis after several days of use, corneal ulceration with prolonged use, and the emergence of resistant bacterial strains have decreased their usefulness for the treatment of bacterial conjunctivitis [2, 18, 23]. Fourth generation fluoroquinolones such as gatifloxacin, moxifloxacin, and besifloxcin are potent, bactericidal, broad-spectrum, and effective against various drug-resistant strains, such as MRSA [1, 2, 51]. They are particularly useful in children who wear contact lens because these children have a higher chance of pseudomonas conjunctivitis

[23]. Fourth generation fluoroquinolones have potent inhibitory activities against both bacterial DNA gyrase (topoisomerase II) and topoisomerase IV which are essential enzymes involved in bacterial DNA replication, transcription, repair, and recombination [1, 38]. As such, the use of these medications is associated with a lower incidence of bacterial resistance [52, 53]. It has been shown that moxifloxacin and besifloxcin achieve the highest mean concentrations in conjunctival tissue and have very favorable pharmacokinetic/pharmacodynamic characteristics [1]. Currently, the fourth generation fluoroquinolones are the drugs of choice for the treatment of bacterial conjunctivitis in childhood whereas the older preparations of ciprofloxacin, ofloxacin, norfloxacin are less commonly used [18, 48]. The recommended dose is one drop in the affected eye twice a day [52, 54]. Ophthalmic fluoroquinolones have minimal ocular adverse effects but are more expensive than other available options [2].

For neonates who have received antibiotic at birth and who do not have acute profuse purulent discharge, the conjunctivitis can best be treated with topical antibiotic, with the exception of topical aminoglycosides and sulfacetamide, for at least 5 to 7 days [42]. Topical aminoglycosides and sulfacetamide are best avoided because of the weak coverage of conjunctival pathogens in the neonatal period [42].

Neonates who have not received antibiotic at birth and who do have acute profuse purulent discharge should be treated with parenteral ceftriaxone (125 mg for term infants and 25 to 50 mg/kg [not to exceed 125 mg] for preterm and low-birth weight infants) for presumptive gonococcal conjunctivitis [13, 42]. Topical antibiotic is unnecessary but may be added to the treatment regimen to reduce the degree of copious purulent discharge [13]. Frequent lavage of the conjunctival fornices with normal saline solution is recommended to remove the inflammatory exudate [13]. For chlamydial conjunctivitis, oral macrolide coupled with topical erythromycin ointment are the treatment of choice and should be given for at least 14 days [43]. For venereal conjunctivitis, the parents should be evaluated and treated if necessary.

Oral antibiotics should be considered for purulent conjunctivitis resistant to treatment with topical antibiotics. Refractory purulent conjunctivitis is often due to penicillin-resistant pneumococcus or *S. aureus*. The oral antibiotics of choice are clindamycin and trimethoprim/sulfamethoxazole [42].

REFERENCES

[1] Benitez-del-Castillo, J., Verboven, Y., Stroman, D., et al. The role of topical moxifloxacin, a new antibacterial in Europe, in the treatment of bacterial conjunctivitis. *Clin. Drug Investig.* 2011;31:543-557.

[2] Chang, M.H., Fung, H.B. Topical fluoroquinolone for the treatment of bacterial conjunctivitis. *Clin. Ther.* 2010;32:454-471.

[3] Mah, F. Bacterial conjunctivitis in pediatrics and primary care. *Pediatr. Clin. North Am.* 2006;53(Suppl 1):7-10.

[4] Rose, P. Management strategies for acute infective conjunctivitis in primary care: a systematic review. *Expert Opin. Pharmacother.* 2007;8:1903-1921.

[5] Smith, A.F., Waycaster, C. Estimate of the direct and indirect annual cost of bacterial conjunctivitis in the United States. *BMC. Ophthalmol.* 2009;9:13.

[6] Azari, A.A., Barney, N.P. Conjunctivitis: a systematic review of diagnosis and treatment. *JAMA.* 2013;310:1721-1729.

[7] Fitch, C.P., Rapoza, P.A.,Owens, S., et al. Epidemiology and diagnosis of acute conjunctivitis at an inner-city hospital. *Ophthalmology.* 1989;96:1215-1220.

[8] Gigliotti, F., Williams, W.T., Hayden, F.G., et al. Etiology of acute conjunctivitis in children. *J. Pediatr.* 1981;98:531-536.

[9] Pichichero, M.E. Bacterial conjunctivitis in children: antibacterial treatment options in an era of increasing drug resistance. *Clin. Pediatr.* 2011;50:7-13.

[10] Høvding, G. Acute bacterial conjunctivitis. Acute bacterial conjunctivitis. *Acta Ophthalmol.* 2008;86:5-17.

[11] Gul, S.S., Jamal, M., Khan, N. Ophthalmia neonatorum. *J. Coll. Physicians. Surg. Pak.* 2010;20:595-598.

[12] Darville, T. *Chlamydia trachomatis* infections in neonates and young children. *Semin. Pediatr. Infect. Dis.* 2005;16:235-244.

[13] Richards, A., Guzman-Cottrill, J.A. Conjunctivitis. *Pediatr. Rev.* 2010;31:196-208.

[14] Cronau, H., Kankanala, R.R., Mauger, T. Diagnosis and management of red eye in primary care. *Am. Fam. Physician.* 2010;81:137-144.

[15] Epling, J. Bacterial conjunctivitis. *Clin. Evid. (Online).* 2012 Feb 20;2012. pii 704.

[16] Patel, P.B., Diaz, M.C., Bennett, J.E., et al. Clinical features of bacterial conjunctivitis in children. *Acad. Emerg. Med.* 2007;14:1-5.

[17] Wagner, R.S., Aquino, M. Pediatric ocular inflammation. *Immunol. Allergy Clin. North Am.* 2008;28:169-188.

[18] Meaders, B.C., Azar, J.M. Bacterial conjunctivitis: a review of therapies and approaches. *Adv. NPs. PAs.* 2012;3:25-29, 34.

[19] Mueller, J.B., McStay, C.M. Ocular infection and inflammation. *Emerg. Med. Clin. North Am.* 2008;26:57-72.

[20] Alter, S.J., Vidwan, N.K., Sobande, P.O., et al. Common childhood bacterial infections. *Curr. Probl. Pediatr. Adolesc. Health Care.* 2011;41:256-283.

[21] Leung, A.K. Sticky eye. In: Jones, R., Britten, N., Culpepper, L. (eds). *Oxford Textbook of Primary Medical Care.* Oxford: Oxford University Press; 2004, pp.1087-1089.

[22] Meltzer, J.A., Kunkov, S., Crain, E.F. Identifying children at low risk for bacterial conjunctivitis. *Arch. Pediatr. Adolesc. Med.* 2010;164:263-267.

[23] Sethuraman, U., Kamat, D. The red eye: evaluation and management. *Clin. Pediatr.* 2009;48:588-600.

[24] Bodor, F.F. Systemic antibiotics for treatment of the conjunctivitis-otitis media syndrome. *Pediatr. Infect. Dis. J.* 1989;8:287-290.

[25] Wadhwani, M., D'souza, P., Jain, R., et al. Conjunctivitis in the newborn - a comparative study. *Indian J. Pathol. Microbiol.* 2011;54:254-257.

[26] Baynham, J.T., Moorman, M.A., Donnellan, C., et al. Antibacterial effect of human milk for common causes of paediatric conjunctivitis. *Br. J. Ophthalmol.* 2013;97:377-379.

[27] Everts, R.J., Barnett, T., Lahood, B.R. The utility of routine conjunctival swabs in management of conjunctivitis. *N. Z. Med. J.* 2011;124:64-71.

[28] Wong, A.H., Barg, S.S., Leung, A.K. Seasonal and perennial allergic conjunctivitis. *Recent Pat. Inflamm. Allergy Drug Discov.* (in press)

[29] Ono, S.J., Abelson, M.B. Allergic conjunctivitis: update on pathophysiology and prospects for future treatment. *J. Allergy. Clin. Immunol.* 2005;115(1):118-122.

[30] Leung, A.K., Bowen, T.J. Seasonal allergic rhinitis and food allery. In: Bergman, A.B. ed. *Twenty Common Problems in Pediatrics.* New York: McGraw-Hill, 2001, pp.219-233.

[31] Leung, A.K., Hon, K.L. Seasonal allergic rhinitis. *Recent Pat. Inflamm. Allergy Drug Discov.* 2013;17:187-201.

[32] Leung, A.K., Hon, K.L. *Atopic Dermatitis: a review for the Primary Care Physician.* New York: Nova Science Publishers, Inc., 2012, pp1-113.

[33] Bielory, B.P., O'Brien, T.P., Bielory, L. Management of seasonal allergic conjunctivitis: guide to therapy. *Acta Ophthalmol.* 2012;90(5):399-407.

[34] Tarlan, B., Kiratli, H. Subconjunctival hemorrhage: risk factors and potential indicators. *Clin. Ophthalmol.* 2013;7:1163-1170.

[35] Visscher, K.L., Hutnik, C.M., Thomas, M. Evidence-based treatment of acute infective conjunctivitis: breaking the cycle of antibiotic prescribing. *Can. Fam. Physician.* 2009;55:1071-1075.

[36] Selmi, C. Diagnosis and classification of autoimmune uveitis. *Autoimmun. Rev.* 2014;Jan 12. pii:S1568-9972(14)00018-4. doi: 10.1016/j.autrev.2014.01.006.[Epub ahead of print]

[37] Leung, A.K. Kawaski disease. In: Leung, A.K. (ed). *Common Problems in Ambulatory Pediatrics: Specific Clinical Problems*, volume 1. New York: Nova Science Publishers, Inc., 2011, pp.379-384.

[38] Keating, G.M. Moxifloxacin 0.5% ophthalmic solution in bacterial conjunctivitis. *Drugs.* 2011;7:89-99.

[39] Bertino, J.S., Zhang, J.Z. Besifloxacin, a new ophthalmic fluoroquinolone for the treatment of bacterial conjunctivitis. *Expert Opin. Pharmcother.* 2009;10:2545-2554.

[40] Sheikh, A., Hurwitz, B. Antibiotics versus placebo for acute bacterial conjunctivitis. *Cochrane Database Syst. Rev.* 2006; Issue 2: CD001211. doi:10.1002/14651858. CD001211.pub2.

[41] Sheikh, A., Hurwitz, B. Antibiotics versus placebo for acute bacterial conjunctivitis. *Cochrane Database Syst. Rev.* 2012; Issue 9: CD001211. doi:10.1002/14651858. CD001211.pub3.

[42] Block, S.L. Etiologic and therapeutic pitfalls of newborn conjunctivitis. *Pediatr. Ann.* 2012;41:310-313.

[43] Zuppa, A.A., D'Andrea, V., Catenazzi, P., et al. Ophthalmia neonatorum: what kind of prophylaxis? *J. Matern. Fetal Neonatal Med.* 2011;24:769-773.

[44] Editorial. Management of acute infective conjunctivitis. *Drug Ther. Bull.* 2011;49:78-81.

[45] Ohnsman, C.M. Exclusion of students with conjunctivitis from school: policies of state departments of health. *J. Pediatr. Ophthalmol.* 2007;44:101-105.

[46] Doona, M., Walsh, J.B. Use of chloramphenicol as topical eye medication: time to cry halt. *BMJ.* 1995;310:1217-1218.

[47] Doshi, B., Sarkar, S. Topical administration of chloramphenicol can induce acute hepatitis. *BMJ.* 2009;338:b1699. DOI: 10.1136/bmj.b1699.

[48] Golde, K.T., Gardiner, M.F. Bacterial conjunctivitis in children: a current review of pathogens and treatment. *Int. Ophthalmol. Clin.* 2011;51:85-92.

[49] Bremond-Gignac, D., Mariani-Kurkdjian, P., Beresniak, A., et al. Efficacy and safety of azithromycin 1.5% eye drops for purulent bacterial conjunctivitis in pediatric patients. *Pediatr. Infect. Dis. J.* 2010;29:222-226.

[50] Garnock-Jones, K.P. Azithromycin 1.5% ophthalmic solution in purulent bacterial or trachomatous conjunctivitis. *Drugs*. 2012;72:361-373.

[51] Comstock, T.L., Paterno, M.R., DeCory, H.H., et al. Safety and tolerability of besifloxacin ophthalmic suspension 0.6% in the treatment of bacterial conjunctivitis. Data from six clinical and phase I safety studies. *Clin. Drug Investig*. 2010;30:675-685.

[52] DeLeon, J., Silverstein, B.E., Allaire, C., et al. Besifloxacin ophthalmic suspension 0.6% administered twice daily for 3 days in the treatment of bacterial conjunctivitis in adults and children. *Clin. Drug Investig.* 2012;32:303-317.

[53] Hass, W., Gearinger, L.S., Hesje, C.K., et al. Microbiological etiology and susceptibility of bacterial conjunctivitis isolates from clinical trials with ophthalmic, twice-daily besifloxacin. *Adv. Ther.* 2012;29:442-455.

[54] Tauber, S., Cupp, G., Garber, R., et al. Microbiological efficacy of a new ophthalmic formulation of moxifloxacin dosed twice-daily for bacterial conjunctivitis. *Adv. Ther.* 2010;28:566-574.

In: Conjunctivitis
Editor: Elias H. Bazile

ISBN: 978-1-63321-621-1

Chapter 5

HEMORRHAGIC CONJUNCTIVITIS: EPIDEMIOLOGICAL, CLINICAL AND VIROLOGICAL FINDINGS FROM 45 YEARS OF STUDY

Magilé de la Caridad Fonseca Quintana*
and Luis Sarmiento Pérez#
Enterovirus Disease Laboratory, Virology Department.
Pedro Kourí Tropical
Medicine Institute, Havana, Cuba
Cellular Autoimmunity Unit, Department of Clinical Sciences,
Skåne University
Hospital, Lund University, Malmo, Sweden

ABSTRACT

Acute hemorrhagic conjunctivitis is characterized by the rapid onset of severely painful conjunctivitis and subconjunctival hemorrhage. Coxsackievirus A24 variant and Enterovirus 70 are the major etiological agents involved in acute hemorrhagic conjunctivitis. The first outbreak of acute hemorrhagic conjunctivitis was described in 1969 in Ghana, West Africa. A second focus appeared in Java (Indonesia) in 1969-70. Since

* Magilé C Fonseca: magile@ipk.sld.cu
# Luis Sarmiento: lrsarmientop@gmail.com

then, both viruses have spread to five continents in a pandemic fashion over 45 years and are now an important world public health problem. This chapter provides a state-of-the-art review of the major aspects of the etiology, diagnosis, and clinical management and control measures of acute hemorrhagic conjunctivitis.

ACUTE HEMORRHAGIC CONJUNCTIVITIS – OVERVIEW

Acute hemorrhagic conjunctivitis (AHC) was a newly described disease in the 1970s associated with emergence of enterovirus 70 (EV-70) and coxsackievirus A24 variant (CV-A24v). Since the first reports from Ghana in 1969, subsequent epidemics of AHC have continued in various locations throughout the world [1-5].

EV-70 and CV-A24v are small, non-enveloped, single-stranded, positive-sense RNA viruses from the enterovirus genus in the family Picornaviridae. The original classification of human enteroviruses has been substituted by a taxonomic scheme based on molecular and biological properties of the viruses. This revised classification recognizes at least 12 species, however; only 4 species (A-D) affects humans. CV-A24v and EV-70 belong to distinct human enterovirus subgroups, human enterovirus C (HEC) and human enterovirus D (HED), respectively [6].

The lack of a lipid envelope contributes to the structural stability of the CV-A24v and EV-70 in the external and host environment, including in exposure to human gastric acid. CV-A24v and EV-70 are stable in liquid media and they can survive in water, organic liquids, sewage, surface and fomites for several days. At -70° C, infectivity persists for many years whereas at 4° C, it persists for weeks. The infectious virus is relatively resistant to many common laboratory disinfectants, including 70% ethanol, isopropanol, dilute lysol, and quaternary ammonium compounds. The viruses are also resistant to lipid solvents, including ether and chloroform but they can be inactivated by formaldehyde, gluteraldehyde, strong acid, sodium hypochlorite, and free residual chlorine. Concentration, pH, extraneous organic materials, and contact time affects the degree of inactivation by these compounds [7].

AHC may result from direct inoculation of via hand to eye contact, unlike most other enteroviral diseases that first require replication in the intestine, before spreading to the target organ. Thus, CV-A24v and EV-70 spread mostly by direct or indirect contact with eye secretions [4, 13]. Since the human conjunctiva is the primary site of virus infection and multiplication, AHC usually develops within 24 hours after exposure. The AHC incubation period is estimated to be 12 to 72 hours. The disease is self-limiting; the symptoms subside rapidly, usually by the third day. Recovery is complete within the following week, even in the absence of any treatment [3-5, 8-13].

Although the specimen with the highest sensitivity for establishing an acute infection is a specimen of conjunctival swabs, it is possible to detect both viruses in the respiratory or stool specimen. Emerging evidences suggest that replication and infection of EV-70 in the gastrointestinal tract typically occurs in very short periods. In contrast, CV-A24v is frequently associated with respiratory disease. Thus, while the eye-hand-fomite seems to be the main route of transmission, respiratory and fecal-conjunctival transmission may also occur. Accordingly, it is reasonable to assume that both route of transmission could explain the high transmission rate of the disease [4, 13-22].

The humoral immune responses to AHC viruses are transient, weak or undetectable. The post epidemic decline in seropositive individuals is thought to be associated with the recurrence of AHC epidemics [8, 23-25]. Overall the antibody levels markedly decreased every year. Consequently, most of the patients who had AHC will not have resistance against reinfection 5-7 years after the initial infection.

This fact might also explain the widespread transmission of this viruses and the occurrence of large epidemics [8, 26, 27].

The prevalence of AHC is not influenced by sex or race. However, data from many AHC outbreaks suggest a higher attack rate among males than among females. Epidemic hemorrhagic conjunctivitis is prevalent in all age groups but children aged 2-10 years are at highest risk [8, 32].

The epidemiology of AHC disease is characterized by explosive outbreaks in densely populated areas where promiscuity is large and poor hygiene, usually during warm and humid weather periods. Indeed, tropical and subtropical developing coastal countries and nearly all such regions of the world have been affected [8, 28].

Numerous outbreaks of acute hemorrhagic conjunctivitis due to CV-A24v have occurred periodically over two consecutive years with isolated strains clustered in the same lineage [22, 29-31]. It is important to note that although CV-A24 variant and EV-70 are the major etiological agent involved in AHC, a taxonomically diverse group of viruses such as the Newcastle disease virus and certain Adenovirus may cause conjunctival hemorrhages. In addition Chlamydia, bacteria and amoebae are reported to cause conjunctival hemorrhages [8].

EV-70 Chronological Review

Acute hemorrhagic conjunctivitis suddenly emerged in an eastern suburb of Accra, the capital of Ghana in West Africa, in 1969. It was nicknamed locally "Apollo 11 disease" because it coincided with the time of the Apollo 11 landing on the moon. It spread like wildfire along the south-eastward and north-westerly Africa and reached epidemic proportions in the Mediterranean coast of North Africa [1, 2]. Another focus of AHC was established in South East Asia (Indonesia, Singapore, Cambodia, Philippines, Vietnam) Japan and India, but it was not until 1971 when Kono and collaborators identified the EV-70 as one of the two etiological agents responsible for those outbreaks. Thus, between 1969 and 1974, EV-70 showed an emerging period characterized by limited spreading particularly in tropical and subtropical coast areas in the Eastern hemisphere. Small outbreaks were also reported in Europe (England, France, Russia and Yugoslavia) [8, 33, 34].

It was not until the early 1980s, however, that America and Australia were affected in the second worldwide pandemic. The first cases in the Western hemisphere occurred in Brazil and then, the disease spread to the north of South America, the Caribbean Islands, Central America and the United States (Florida and North Carolina). Other epidemics in Nigeria, Zaire, India and Pakistan occurred in the same time period.

To date, no EV-70 epidemic has been reported since the last reports from Israel, Saudi Arabia, India, the Caribbean Islands and Japan, in the 1990s [35-37].

The question of the origin of the virus remains discussed considering the way in which the pandemic arose. Kono concluded that a new disease has become apparent, possibly from a single focus in Africa. A reasonable explanation for this conclusion done by Kono could be the adaptation of an animal virus to man. Indeed, serological evidence suggests the occurrence of infections in animals with a virus resembling that of acute hemorrhagic conjunctivitis [33, 38].

Another important observation is the fact that phylogenetic studies of different strains isolated during epidemics have shown that the number of base changes of isolates became greater as the years elapsed. In addition, the number of base changes among recent isolates from different areas of the world was much greater than those among early isolates. The time of emergence of the original strain it was estimated to be around August 1967 +/- 15 months. From the results, it has been hypothesized that EV-70 may have emerged from a single common ancestor. Thus, the virus branched into many strains early during the first pandemic and has evolved in a divergent fashion, yielding genetically polymorphic viruses in the world [39, 40].

CV-A24v Chronological Review

An AHC epidemic in Singapore in 1970 and in subsequent epidemics in Hong Kong and Malaysia, a new strain of the Coxsackievirus A24 (CV-A24v) was incriminated as the cause of the pandemic [3]. In contrast to the rapid and wide spread of EV-70, CV-A24v was long restricted to Southeast Asia. Not until the mid-1980s was the Far East affected. Epidemics in other Asian countries, including Taiwan, Korea and Japan occurred 15 years after the initial outbreak in South Asia. AHC caused by CV-A24v was first detected in Africa (Tunisia, Congo, Angola, Ghana, and Nigeria) and the Western hemisphere in 1986 where the epidemic started from South America (Brazil) and reached the Caribbean Islands, Central America and the United States [20, 28, 35, 42].

A silent period during the 1990s was characterized by only a few outbreaks reported in Pakistan, Tunisia, Taiwan in 1993-1994, Thailand 1992, and China 1998 (27). However, further reports of wide AHC outbreaks were described from the Caribbean including Saint Croix, Antigua/Barbuda, Bahamas, British Virgin Islands, St. Christopher/ Nevis, Trinidad and Tobago, Suriname and Cuba (1992-1993, 1997) [20, 28, 42].

In the 2000s, a reemerging period has been characterized by extremely rapid spread throughout the world. Reemerging outbreaks of AHC occurred in Southern China, Korea, Malaysia, Nepal, Tunisia, Guiana, Guadeloupe West India, Congo, Morocco, Pakistan, Singapore, Taiwan and Spain. The disease was expanded once again to the South America (Brazil) and extended to the Caribbean Islands (Puerto Rico 2003, French Guiana and West Indies). It is noteworthy that two epidemic stages have been experienced Taiwan (2000-2002, 2006-2007), Cuba (2003, 2008-2009), Brazil (2003, 2009) where phylogenetic analyses suggests that the viruses have been independently introduced in each epidemic period [20, 28, 43].

It is important to notice that previous phylogenetic studies of the CA24v genome have revealed three genotypes (GI-GIII) derived from a common ancestor which time of emergence was estimated to be November, 1963 +/- 21 months. Genotypes I and II include the isolates obtained in Singapore, Hong Kong and Thailand during the 1970s. Genotype III comprises six clusters of strains isolated from Asia, Pakistan and Ghana from 1985 to 1994 [30].

Remarkably, a new genotype (GIV) was recently identified based on the same analysis. Genotype IV is divided into three clusters (GIV-C1, GIV-C2 and GIV-C3) and includes recent strains isolated from South Korea, China, India, Guadeloupe and African countries (Congo, Guiana and Morocco) and the Western Hemisphere [27, 40].

DIAGNOSTIC

As has been noted elsewhere, AHC usually occurs in epidemics with a high rate of transmission.

Thus, AHC is a major public health problem, particularly in heavily populated areas. The rapid identification of the causative agent is required to implement proper public health measures to limit the extension of the outbreak [33, 35, 45]. The ocular symptoms caused by EV-70 and CV-A24v are clinically indistinguishable and constitute the AHC syndrome. Therefore, AHC should be used as the term representing an enteroviral eye disease characterized by the AHC syndrome.

Historically the identification of the AHC serotypes has been based on virus isolation from conjunctival swab inoculated onto human cell lines [8, 12, 13, 19-22].

Remarkably, ongoing studies from our group are starting to unveil the contribution of rectal swabs and feces as a good source for viral detection. Accumulative data indicate that HeLa and Hep-2 have been the cells lines most widely used for the CV-A24v isolation [34]. However, the frequency of CV-A24v isolation positivity is not entirely defined by the used cell line [19].

Because changes in cell morphology (e.g., cell rounding followed by the shrinkage and degeneration of the cell sheet) are not specific for any virus group, a confirmatory assay is needed for further typing of an isolated virus strain. Viral isolates are then confirmed by neutralization assay, electron microscopic, serological tests or immunofluorescence using monoclonal antibodies specific.

However, classical virus isolation and identification remains difficult and time-consuming [45, 46]. Recently, new approaches such as the use the extraction kits (manual or automatically), RT-PCR and RT-PCR in real time assays, using generic or specific primers; sequence analysis of structural (VP1, VP2, VP4) and non-structural regions (3C,3D) with their respective phylogenetic analysis; commercially developed (Amplicor Enterovirus PCR) kits and another news technologies have documented an extremely rapid, sensitive and specific diagnostic modality for the detection of an enterovirus in clinical specimens or tissue culture [44-53].

Clinical Management

Since the conjunctiva is directly exposed to the external environment, it is therefore endangered by a multitude of antigens and pathogenic microorganisms. It is well known that conjunctiva, as a mucosa, is protected by the mucosal immune system that uses innate and adaptive effect or mechanisms present in the tissue [54]. However, it is an immuneprivileged site, because the T-cell response in this area is suppressed [55]. This protects the eye from potentially destructive immune responses but also makes defense against infectious agents difficult, especially where T-cell responses are important for immunological defense [56]. Therefore, viral infection is the most common cause of conjunctivitis and they are estimated to account for 80% of all cases of acute conjunctivitis. It is notable that the rate of clinical accuracy in diagnosing viral conjunctivitis is less than 50% compared to laboratory confirmation [57, 58].

Most viral infections produce a mild, self-limiting conjunctivitis that may heal within a few weeks, and can affect all ages. Signs include normal vision, normal pupil size and reaction to light; diffuse conjunctival injections (redness), preauricular lymphadenopathy, lymphoid follicle on the undersurface of the eyelid. Symptoms are characterized by mild to no pain, diffuse hyperemia, occasional gritty discomfort with mild itching, watery to serous discharge, photophobia, often unilateral at onset with second eye involved within one or two days. However, AHC is characterized by the sudden onset of hyperemic conjunctiva, subconjunctival hemorrhages, chemosis, lid swelling, tearing, photophobia, and severe pain. [3-5, 8-12, 58].

Under normal conditions, the cornea is highly resistant to viral invasion. However, when epithelial integrity is breached, virus may invade the cornea, resulting in infectious keratitis. Thus, inflammation of the conjunctiva can also occur in combination with corneal inflammation and subepithelial infiltrates, causing severe keratoconjunctivitis, which is one of the leading causes of visual impairment and blindness. There are usually no other systemic symptoms or as rarely to frequently occurring upper respiratory illness (nasopharyngitis, coryza), malaise, fever, headache, dizziness and/or gastrointestinal illness. However, neurological complications associated to EV-70 infections such as transient lumbar radiculomyelopathy and poliomyelitis-like illness were reported 2-4 weeks after conjunctivitis. EV-70 is neurotropic and approximately 1:10,000 AHC patients, usually males 20-40 years of age, have mild to permanent weakness in the muscles of the face and/or extremities [3-5, 8-13].

Now, however, it is known that the clinical signs can change from one outbreak to another. Perhaps, one of the most illustrative examples of this phenomenon is the enteroviral conjunctivitis in Taiwan which displayed several distinct outbreaks over an 18-year period (59).

There were four epidemics of EV-70 AHC in 1980-1981 and 1983-1984 [60]. Epidemics of AHC caused by CV-A24v occurred in Taiwan in 2000–2002 and 2006–2007 following the four initial epidemics in 1985–1986, 1988–1989, 1990–1991 and 1994 [27]. Subconjunctival hemorrhage occurred in CV-A24v conjunctivitis with an incidence of 44.1% (63/143 patients) in the 1985–1986 outbreaks, and 46.4% (52/112 patients) in the 1988–1989 outbreaks, whereas the incidence increased to 71.6% (53/74 patients) in the 1990–1991 outbreaks and 78.2% (45/55 patients) in the 1994 outbreaks [59]. The severity of the AHC in 1989 was found to be milder than the AHC associated with CV-A24v in 1985.

However, the AHC presented more severe signs, especially subconjunctival hemorrhage, in the 1990s outbreaks than in those during the 1980s. Strikingly, only two amino acid differences were commonly identified in the isolates after 1985 [29, 61].

More interesting, the severity of ocular symptoms and signs observed in 2000–2002 was milder than that in other outbreaks, however, strains isolated during 2006–2007 showed the same patterns of amino acid residue changes as those isolated in 2000–2001 [27].

On the other hand, two outbreaks of AHC caused by CV-A24v were reported in Cuba during 2008 and 2009. Phylogenetic analysis of the 3Cpro region revealed that Cuban strains isolated during 2008–2009 outbreaks had highest nucleotide identity with CV-A24v strains isolated from outbreaks of hemorrhagic conjunctivitis in Taiwan 2006–2007. It is notable that, although three amino acid changes were found in the strains isolated in 2009, no differences in clinical signs and symptoms were noticed in both years and it did not differ from those previously reported in Taiwan during the 2006-2007 outbreaks [19].

Therefore it is difficult to tell whether the genomic alteration of viruses or a change in host immune response may explain the fluctuation of the patient's clinical signs among epidemics. Thus, the role of amino acid substitution in modifying clinical symptoms remains to be solved. Comparative studies on pathogenic differences of parallel variants from relevant virus strains may reveal the amino acids and/or nucleotides of the virus genome, which are the most critical for aggravation of conjunctivitis symptoms.

Prevention and Treatment

It's been noted that viral conjunctivitis, especially AHC, is highly contagious. Thus, secondary attack rates in households with (initial) single patients are extremely high. Therefore, the most important step in management of AHC conjunctivitis is prevention of transmission [62].

Since the viruses spreads through direct contact via contaminated fingers, medical instruments, swimming pool water, or personal items; patient education and good hygiene are important in decreasing the spread of acute viral conjunctivitis. The patients should be counseled to practice strict hand washing and avoid sharing personal items [63]. In addition, patients should be kept from school or work until there is no discharge [64]. In a study from China, authors assessed the efficacy of a quarantine method to help control outbreaks of AHC in schools. It was estimated that without intervention, almost all students would have become infected in 23 days. This suggests that quarantine programs could be used to curtail AHC outbreaks at schools and reduce the number of accumulated cases [65].

Thus, early recognition and identification of AHC are critical for successful response. We therefore recommend that state and local public health agencies in tropical areas where AHC is common to develop capacity to better ensure prompt clinical diagnosis and laboratory detection of this disease. These scenarios highlight the value of physician awareness of the signs, symptoms, and diagnostic testing's related to AHC. Once AHC is detected, no delay should occur in telling the public about the outbreak or in disseminating strategies to minimize the dissemination. In addition, public messaging should also provide specific actions that members of the public can take to protect themselves, their families, and their communities.

For example, in an outbreak of CV-A24v-associated AHC that took place in Cuba during 2008-2009, control measures implemented at the time of discovery of the outbreak were critical to mitigate the outbreak [19]. Once the outbreak was confirmed, health officials undertook education efforts including disseminating public health information by press release, radio and TV messages. Other measures included encouraging careful and frequent hand washing; avoiding sharing towels, bedding, makeup and other personal items to prevent transmission from potential fomite sources. This effort also included the implementation of conservative measures such as supportive and symptomatic treatment at home under the supervision of the family doctor for these patients [19].

In contrast, delayed detection and institution of preventive measures during an outbreak of viral conjunctivitis in military occurred in 2005 in Singapore were associated with delayed effectiveness of the control measures. Every delay in outbreak detection by one day resulted in a delay in terminating the outbreak by 0.82 days ($p = 0.01$) [66]. Lessons learned during these outbreaks also highlight the need for ongoing surveillance for AHC, especially as decreases in funding for these activities are anticipated.

It is important to notice that though the symptoms may be addressed; neither preventive nor therapeutic treatment is currently available. To date, treatment is supportive and may include cold compresses and ocular decongestants. Treatment with topical steroids should not be used because of the risk of corneal perforation and microbial superinfection of the cornea [67].

Various agents such as Benzimidazole compounds (Enviradone and Enviroxime), Arildone or interferon have been shown to inhibit enterovirus replication, but none are available as chemotherapeutics agents [68].

Indeed, separate research groups have described that natural human interferons (IFN) or recombinant human IFNs (rIFN-alpha and rIFN-beta) are effective in inhibiting CV-A24v infection in human conjunctival cell cultures. However, the antiviral activity of IFN against acute hemorrhagic conjunctivitis in vivo may vary with the CV-A24v isolates, the multiplicity of infections, the type of IFN, and the time of infection with respect to beginning IFN treatment. In addition there are reports that failed to observe a beneficial effect of IFNs [69-71].

On the other hand, in vitro studies have indicated that Arildone can inhibit AHC viruses. In these studies the inhibitory effects of combination of Arildone and IFN were shown to be additive. Other studies reports that Enviradone and Enviroxime can inhibit AHC viruses in vitro at concentrations that are not cytotoxic, which suggest that Enviradone and Enviroxime may prove to be useful against AHC [72, 73].

However, data on antiviral agents targeting RNA viruses as causes of conjunctivitis are mostly limited to animal and in vitro studies and there have been no studies about the efficacy of these compounds against AHC in vivo. Thus, novel antiviral strategies are urgently needed.

Since viruses are obligate intracellular parasites that rely on the host organism for successful replication and subsequent particle packaging and release, the organisms have evolved various defense mechanisms to combat viral infection. Recent advances have revealed that RNA interference (RNAi) has emerged as an integral and critical component of antiviral defense [74]. RNAi can suppress gene expression at the transcriptional level, however, RNAi most often act post transcriptionally to destabilize and/or inhibit the translation of complementary target mRNAs in a sequence-specific manner. These properties confer unparalleled specificity and precision to RNAi-mediated gene silencing as an effective antiviral mechanism [75, 76].

One of the most representative studies evaluating the the use of small-interfering RNA (siRNA) molecules for replication inhibition of CV-A24v and EV-70 was reported by Jun and their collaborators in 2008 and 2011. These researchers showed that siRNAs targeting a conserved genome region of CV-A24 can possess universally effective anti- CV-A24v activity in conjunctival cells, as well as HeLa cells. The same group of researcher developed a novel siRNA that targeted a conserved region of both EV-70 and CV-A24v, which was able to decrease replication and protein synthesis of both of the viruses in MRC5 and primary human conjunctival cells [77, 78]. In addition Tan et al demonstrated a significant reduction of EV-70 replication in the RD cell line treated with chemically synthesized siRNAs prior to and after EV-70 infection [79].

Taken together, these data highlight the potential of siRNA as a prophylactic and therapeutic intervention approach against viruses-causing AHC. Use of this siRNA may therefore be clinically feasible in the treatment of patients with AHC. For siRNA-based agents to achieve therapeutic benefits in clinical settings, a safe and effective siRNA delivery system is needed [80]. However, in a mouse model of respiratory syncytial virus (RSV) infection of the eye, synthetic anti-RSV siRNA, applied topically shortly before viral inoculation, prevented spread of infection in the eye and lung [81]. Accordingly, if an effective level of siRNA can be topically transported into conjunctival cells, it may have therapeutic effects against AHC in vivo.

Further studies are needed to define the therapeutic efficacy of siRNA against viruses responsible for the development of AHC which will open new prospects for prevention and therapy.

REFERENCES

[1] Chatterjee S, Quarcoopome CO, Apenteng A. Unusual type of epidemic conjunctivitis in Ghana. *Br. J. Ophthalmol.* 1970; 54:628-30.

[2] Kono R, Sasagawa A, Ishii K, Siginra S, Ochi M, Matsumya H, et al. Pandemic of new type of conjunctivitis. *Lancet* 1972; 1: 1191-94.

[3] Lim KH, Yin-Murphy M. An epidemic of conjunctivitis in Singapore in 1970. *Singapore Med. J.* 1971; 12:247–49.

[4] Mirkovic RR, Kono R, Yin-Murphy M, Sohier R, Schmidt NJ, Melnick, JL. Enterovirus type 70: the etiologic agent of pandemic acute haemorrhagic conjunctivitis. *Bull WHO* 1973; 49:341-46.

[5] Mirkovic RR, Schmidt NJ, Yin-Murphy M, Melnick JL. Enterovirus etiology of the 1970 Singapore epidemic of acute conjunctivitis. *Intervirology* 1974; 4: 119-27.

[6] International Committee on Taxonomy of Viruses (ICTV).2014. http://ictvonline.org/.

[7] Pallansch M y Roos R: Enteroviruses: Polioviruses, Coxsackieviruses, Echoviruses, and Newer Enteroviruses. En: D. M. Knipe y P. M. Howley (eds.). Fields Virology 2007. 5th ed. Philadelphia - New York: Lippincott Williams & Wilkins.

[8] Hierholzer JC, Hilliard KA, Esposito JJ. Serosurvey for acute hemorrhagic conjunctivitis virus (enterovirus 70) antibodies in the Southeastern United States, with review of the literature and some epidemiologic implications. *Am. J. Epidemiol* 1975; 102:533-544.

[9] Kono R, Miyamura K, Tajiri E, Sasagawa A, Phuapradit P, Roogwithu N,Vejjajiva A, Jayavasu C, Thongcharoen P, Wasi C, Rodprassert P. Virological and serological studies of neurological complications of acute haemorrhagic conjunctivitis in Thailand. *J. Infect. Dis.* 1977; 135:706-13.

[10] Wadia, N.H. Neurological manifestations of enterovirus 70: a 15-year review from India. In: Y. Uchida, K. Ishii, K. Miyamura and S. Yamazaki (Eds.), *Acute Hemorrhagic Conjunctivitis; Etiology, Epidemiology and Clinical Manifestations*, 1989. Karger, New York, pp. 251-266.

[11] Higgins PG. Enteroviral conjunctivitis and its neurological complications. *Arch. of Virol.* 1982; 73: 91-101.

[12] Waldman, E. A. Takimoto, S. Ishida, M. A. Kitamura, C. Mendonca, L. I. Enterovirus 70 in the metropolitan region of Sao Paulo, Brazil, from 1984 to 1987: infection aspects in endemic and epidemic periods. *Rev Inst. Med. Trop. Sao Paulo* 1990; 32(3):221-28.

[13] Palacios G and Oberste MS. Enteroviruses as agents of emerging infectious diseases. *Journal of Neuro Virology* 2005, 11: 424–433.

[14] Pallansch MA. Acute hemorrhagic conjunctivitis. In: *Hunter's tropical medicine*. Strickland GT (ed). Philadelphia: WB, Saunders, 2000; 226–27.

[15] Yin-Murphy, M., K. H. Lim, and Y. M. Ho. A coxsackievirus type A24 epidemic of acute conjunctivitis. *Southeast Asian J. Trop. Med.* 1976, 7:1–5.

[16] Yin-Murphy, M., Baharuddin-Ishak, M. C. Phoon, and V. T. Chow. A recent epidemic of Coxsackie virus type A24 acute haemorrhagic conjunctivitis in Singapore. *Br. J. Ophthalmol* 1986.70:869–873.

[17] Wright P W, Strauss GH, and Langford M.Acute hemorrhagic conjunctivitis. *Am. Fam. Physician* 1992, 45:173–178.

[18] Avalos Redon I, Mas Lago PJ, Sarmiento Perez LR, Palomera Puentes RE, Bello Corredor M. Outbreak of Acute hemorrhagic conjunctivitis in Cuba. *Mem. Inst. Oswaldo Cruz* 1999; 94(4):467–8.

[19] Fonseca MC, Sarmiento L, Resik S, Pereda N, Rodríguez H, Kourí V, Martínez PA, Piñón A, Limonta D, Más P, Hung LH. Isolation of Coxsackievirus A24 variant from patients with hemorrhagic conjunctivitis in Cuba, 2008-2009.*J. Clin. Virol* 2012; 53: 77– 81.

[20] Nilsson EC, Jamshidi F, Johansson SM, Oberste MS, Arnberg N. Sialic acid is a cellular receptor for coxsckievirus A24 variant, an emerging virus with pandemic potential. *J. Virol.* 2008; 82(6):3061–8.

[21] Kuo, PC, Lin JY, Chen LC, Fang YT, Cheng Y, Wu HY, et al. Molecular and immuno-cytochemical identification of coxsackievirus A-24 variant from the acute hemorrhagic conjunctivitis in Taiwan in 2007. *Eye* (Lond) 2009; 24(1):131-136.

[22] Christopher S, Theogaraj S, Godbole S, John TJ. An epidemic of acute hemorrhagic conjunctivitis due to coxsackievirus A24. *J. Infect. Dis* 1982; 146(1): 16-19.

[23] Kono, R., Miyamura, E., Tajiri, E., Sasagawa, A., Phuapradit, P., Roongwithu, N., Vejjajiva, A., Jayavasu, C., Thongcharoen, P., Wasi, C., Rodprassert, P. Virological and serological studies of neurological complications of acute hemorrhagic conjunctivitis in Thailand. *J. Infect. Dis* 1977; 135: 706-713.

[24] Langford MP, Barber JC, Sear VEF, Clark SW, Patriarca PA, Onarato IM et al. Virus-specific early appearing neutralizing activity and interferon in tears of patients with acute hemorrhagic conjunctivitis. *Curr. Eye Res* 1985; 4: 233-239.

[25] Aoki, K. and H. Sawada. Long-term observation of neutralization antibody after enterovirus 70 infection. *Jpn. J. Ophthalmol.* 1992; 36(4): 465-468.

[26] Wu D, Ke CW, Mo YL, Sun LM, Li H, Chen QX. Multiple outbreaks of acute hemorrhagic conjunctivitis due to a variant of coxsackievirus A24: Guangdong, China, 2007. *J. Med. Virol.* 2008; 80:1762-1768

[27] Chu PY, Ke GM, Chang CH, Lin JC, Sun CY, Huang WL, et al. Molecular epidemiology of coxsackie A type 24 variant in Taiwan, 2000–2007. *J. Clin. Virol.* 2009; 45(4):285-91.

[28] Ishiko H, Takeda N, Miyamura K, Tanimura M, Yamanaka T, Kasuga K, at al.. Phylogenetic different strains of a variant of coxsackievirus A24 were repeatly introduced but discontinued circulating in Japan. *Arch. Virol* 1992; 126: 179–93.

[29] Lin KH, Wang HL, Sheu MM, Huang WL, Chen CW, Yang CS, at al. Molecular epidemiology of a variant of coxsackievirus A24 in Taiwan: two epidemics caused by phylogenetically distinct viruses from 1985 to 1989. *J. Clin. Microbiol* 1993; 31(5):1160–6.

[30] Moura FEA, Ribeiro DCS, Gurgel N, Da Silva Mendes AC, Tavares FN,Timoteo CNG, et al. Acute haemorrhagic conjunctivitis outbreak in the city of Fortaleza, northeast Brazil. *Br. J. Ophthalmol.* 2006; 90(9): 1091–3.

[31] Sane F, Sauter P, Fronval S, Goffard A, Dewilde A, Hober D. Fruit of the emergence of an enterovirus: acute haemorrhagic conjunctivitis. *Ann. Biol. Clin.* (Paris) 2008; 66(5): 485-492.

[32] Acute haemorrhagic conjunctivitis. *Br. Med. J. (Clin Res Ed)* 1982; 284(6318): 833-834.

[33] Likar M, Likar M, Talanyi-Pfeifer L, Marin J. An outbreak of acute hemorrhagic conjunctivitis in Yugoslavia in 1973. *Pathol. Microbiol.* (Basel) 1975; 42(1): 29-35.

[34] Leveque N, Huguet P, Norder H, Chomel JJ. Enteroviruses responsible for acute hemorrhagic conjunctivitis. *Med. Mal. Infect.* 2010; 40(4): 212-218.

[35] Delgado J. Conjuntivitis Hemorrágica Epidémica en Cuba: Caracterización epidemiológica, cronología y situación actual. 1981-1997. Cuba. MINSAP. Unidad de Análisis y Tendencias en Salud UATS 1997; 2(7). ISSN 108-4338.

[36] MMWR Morb Mortal Wkly Rep. Acute hemorrhagic conjunctivitis-American Samoa. 1982, 31(3): 21-22.

[37] Kono R, Sasagawa A, Yamazaki S, Nakazono N, Minami K, Otatsume S, et al. Seroepidemiologic studies of acute hemorrhagic conjunctivitis virus enterovirus type 70 in West Africa. III. Studies with animal sera from Ghana and Senegal. *Am. J. Epidemiol.* 1981; 114(3): 362-368.

[38] Takeda N, Miyamura K, Ogino T, Natori K, Yamazaki S, Sakurai N, et al. Evolution of enterovirus type 70 : oligonucleotide mapping analysis of RNA genome. *Virology* 1984 ; 134 : 375-88.

[39] Miyamura K, Tanimura M, Takeda N, Kono R, Yamazaki S. Evolution of enterovirus 70 in nature: all isolates were recently derived from a common ancestor. *Arch. Virol.* 1986; 89: 1-14.

[40] Ishiko H, Takeda N, Miyamura K, Kato N, Tanimura M, Lin KH, et al. Phylogenetic analysis of a coxsackievirus A24 variant: the most recent worldwide pandemic was caused by progenies of a virus prevalent around 1981. *Virology* 1992; 187:148-759.

[41] MMWR Morb Mortal Wkly. Acute hemorrhagic conjunctivitis outbreak caused by Coxsackievirus A24-Puerto Rico, 2003. 2004, Rep 53(28): 632-634.

[42] Tavares F., Campos Rde M, Burlandy FM, Fontella R, de Melo MM, da Costa EV, et al. Molecular characterization and phylogenetic study of coxsackievirus A24v causing outbreaks of acute hemorrhagic conjunctivitis (AHC) in Brazil. *PLoS One* 2011; 6(8): e23206.

[43] Lin KH, Chern CL, Chu PY, Chang CH, Wang HL, Sheu MM, et al. Genetic analysis of recent Taiwanese isolates of a variant of coxsackievirus A24. *J. Med. Virol.* 2001; 64(3):269–74.

[44] Xiao XL, Wu H, Li YJ, Li HF, He YQ, Chen G, et al. Simultaneous detection of enterovirus 70 and coxsackievirus A24 variant by multiplex real-time RT-PCR using an internal control. *J. Virol. Methods* 2009; 159(1): 23-28.

[45] Oberste MS, Nix WA, Maher K, Pallansch MA. Improved molecular identification of enteroviruses by RT-PCR and amplicon sequencing. *J. Clin. Virol.* 2003;26,375–377.

[46] Shulman LM, Manor Y, Azar R, Handsher R, Vonsover A, Mendelson E, et al. Identification of a new strain of fastidious enterovirus 70 as the causative agent of an outbreak of hemorrhagic conjunctivitis. *J. Clin. Microbiol.* 1997; 35(8): 2145-2149.

[47] Yang CF, De L, Yang SJ, Gómez JR, Cruz JR, Halloway MA, Pallansch MA, Kew OM. Genotype-specific in vitro amplification of sequences of the wild type 3 polioviruses from México and Guatemala. *Virus. Res.* 1992; 24:277–96.

[48] Kishore J, Isomura S. Detection and differentiation of coxsackievirus A24 variant isolate from an epidemic of acute haemorrhagic conjunctivitis in north India by RT-PCR using a novel primer pair. *Indian J. Med. Res.* 2002; 115:176–83.

[49] Nix WA, Oberste MS, Pallansch MA. Sensitive, seminested PCR amplification of VP1 sequences for direct identification of all enterovirus serotypes from original clinical specimens. *J. Clin. Microbiol.* 2006, 44:2698–2704.

[50] Casas GF, Palacios G, Trallero D, Cisterna MC, Freire and Tenorio A. Molecular Characterization of Human Enteroviruses in Clinical Samples: Comparison Between VP2, VP1, and RNA Polymerase Regions Using RT Nested PCR Assays and Direct Sequencing of Products I. *J. Med. Virol.* 2001; 65:138-148.

[51] Coiras JC, Aguilar ML, Garcia I, Casas and Pérez-Breña. Simultaneous Detection of Fourteen Respiratory Viruses in Clinical Specimens by Two Multiplex Reverse Transcription Nested-PCR Assays M.T. *Journal of Medical Virology* 2004; 72:484-495.

[52] Leveque N, Lahlou Amine I, Tcheng R, Falcon D, Rivat N, Dussart P, et al. Rapid diagnosis of acute hemorrhagic conjunctivitis due to Coxsackievirus A24 variant by real-time one-step RT-PCR. *J. Virol. Methods* 2007; 142:89-94.

[53] Park SW, Lee CS, Jang HC, Kim EC, Oh MD, Choe KW. Rapid identification of the Coxsackievirus A24 variant by molecular serotyping in an outbreak of acute hemorrhagic conjunctivitis. *J. Clin. Microbiol.* 2005; 43:1069–71.

[54] Akpek EK and Gottsch, JD Immune defense at the ocular surface. *Eye* 2003, 17, 949–956.

[55] Newman H, Gooding C. Viral ocular manifestations: a broad overview. *Rev. Med. Virol.* 2013; 23(5):281-94.

[56] Lambiase A, Micera A, Sacchetti M, Mantelli F, Bonini S.Toll-like receptors in ocular surface diseases: overview and new findings. *Clin. Sci.* (Lond); 2011;120(10):441-50.

[57] O'Brien TP, Jeng BH, McDonald M, Raizman MB. Acute conjunctivitis: truth and misconceptions. *Curr. Med. Res. Opin.* 2009;25(8):1953-1961.

[58] Dussart P, Cartet G, Huguet P, Leveque N, Hajjar C, Morvan J, et al. Outbreak of acute hemorrhagic conjunctivitis in French Guiana and West Indies caused by coxsackievirus A24 variant: phylogenetic analysis reveals Asian import. *J. Med. Virol.* 2005; 75:559–65.

[59] Chang CH, Lin KH, Sheu MM, Huang WL, Wang HZ, Chen CW. The change of etiological agents and clinical signs of epidemic viral conjunctivitis over an 18-year period in southern Taiwan. *Graefes Arch. Clin. Exp. Ophthalmol.* 2003;241(7):554-60.

[60] Chen, C. W. 1989. Acute hemorrhagic conjunctivitis due to enterovirus 70 in China (Taiwan), p. 161-166. In K. Ishii, *Y. Am. J. Epidemiol.* 101:383-390.

[61] Lin KH, Sheu MM, Wang HL, Huang WL, Chen CW, Yang CS. Study on some biological and antigenic characteristics of CA24v isolates in Taiwan in 1985–1989. *Kaohsiung J. Med. Sci.* 1994; 10:279–286.

[62] Azari AA, Barney NP. Conjunctivitis: a systematic review of diagnosis and treatment. *JAMA* 2013, 310(16):1721-9.

[63] Azar MJ, Dhaliwal DK, Bower KS, Kowalski RP, Gordon YJ. Possible consequences of shaking hands with your patients with epidemic keratoconjunctivitis. *Am. J. Ophthalmol.* 1996; 121(6):711-712.

[64] Cronau H, Kankanala RR, Mauger T.Diagnosis and management of red eye in primary care *Am. Fam. Physician.* 2010; 81(2):137-44.

[65] Chen TM, Liu RC. Study on the efficacy of quarantine during outbreaks of acute hemorrhagic conjunctivitis outbreaks at schools through the susceptive-infective-quarantine-removal model. *Zhonghua Liu Xing Bing Xue Za Zhi*.2013; 34(1):75-9.

[66] Ong AE, Dashraath P, Lee VJ. Management of enteroviral conjunctivitis outbreaks in the Singapore military in 2005. *Southeast Asian J Trop Med Public Health* 2008; 39(3):398-403.

[67] Morrow GL, Abbott RL. Conjunctivitis. *Am Fam Physician.* 1998; 57(4): 735-746.

[68] Skevaki CL, Galani IE, Pararas MV, Giannopoulou KP, Tsakris A. Treatment of viral conjunctivitis with antiviral drugs. Drugs. 2011 Feb 12;71(3):331-47.

[69] Langford MP, Kadi RM, Ganley JP, Yin-Murphy M. Inhibition of epidemic isolates of coxsackievirus type A 24 by recombinant and natural interferon alpha and interferon beta. *Intervirology* 1988; 29 (6): 320-7.

[70] Langford MP, Orillac R, Chen D, Texada D. Systemic and ocular antibody responses to inactivated acute hemorrhagic conjunctivitis (AHC) virus; enterovirus 70 (EV70). *Ocul. Immunol. Inflamm.* 2003; 11 (3): 197-209.

[71] Langford MP, Villarreal AL, Stanton GJ. Antibody and interferon act synergistically to inhibit enterovirus, adenovirus, and herpes simplex virus infection. *Infect. Immun.* 1983 l; 41 (1): 214-8.

[72] Langford MP, Carr DJ, Yin-Murphy M. Activity of arildone with or without interferon against acute hemorrhagic conjunctivitis viruses in cell culture. *Antimicrob Agents Chemother* 1985; 28 (4): 578-80.

[73] Langford MP, Ball WA, Ganley JP. Inhibition of the enteroviruses that cause acute hemorrhagic conjunctivitis (AHC) by benzimidazoles; enviroxime (LY 122772) and enviradone (LY 127123). *Antiviral. Res.* 1995; 27 (4): 355-65.

[74] Zhou R, Rana TM. RNA-based mechanisms regulating host-virus interactions. *Immunol. Rev.* 2013; 253(1):97-111.

[75] Umbach JL, Cullen BR. The role of RNAi and microRNAs in animal virus replication and antiviral immunity. *Genes. Dev.* 2009; 23:1151–1164.

[76] Ding SW, Voinnet O. Antiviral immunity directed by small RNAs. *Cell* 2007; 130:413–426.

[77] Jun EJ, Nam YR, Ahn J, Tchah H, Joo CH, Jee Y, et al. Antiviral potency of a siRNA targeting a conserved region of coxsackievirus A24. *Biochem. Biophys. Res. Commun.* 2008; 376 (2): 389-94.

[78] Jun EJ, Won MA, Ahn J, Ko A, Moon H, Tchah H, et al. An antiviral small-interfering RNA simultaneously effective against the most prevalent enteroviruses causing acute hemorrhagic conjunctivitis. *Invest. Ophthalmol. Vis. Sci.* 2011; 52 (1): 58-63).

[79] Tan EL, Marcus KF, Poh CL. Development of RNA interference (RNAi) as potential antiviral strategy against enterovirus 70. *J. Med. Virol.* 2008; 80 (6): 1025-32.

[80] Dykxhoorn DM, Palliser D, Lieberman J. The silent treatment: siRNAs as small molecule drugs. *Gene. Ther.* 2006; (13) 541–552.

[81] Bitko V, Musiyenko A, Barik S. Viral infection of the lungs through the eye. *J. Virol.* 2007; 81 (2): 783-90.

In: Conjunctivitis
Editor: Elias H. Bazile
ISBN: 978-1-63321-621-1

Chapter 6

TROPICAL CONJUNCTIVITIS

***Somsri Wiwanitkit*[1] *and Viroj Wiwanitkit*[2]**
[1]Wiwanitkit House, Bangkhae, Bangkok Thailand
[2]Faculty of Medicine, University of Nis, Serbia

ABSTRACT

Conjunctivitis is a common ocular problem that can be seen worldwide and it is still under consideration for global public health. There are many causes of conjunctivitis. The interesting group of conjunctivitis disorders is those found in tropical zone. There are many tropical infections and disorders that can induce conjunctivitis and those problems are called tropical conjunctivitis. In this short article, the authors will summarize and discuss on important kinds of tropical conjunctivitis focusing on diagnosis and management.

INTRODUCTION

Conjunctivitis is a common ocular problem that can be seen worldwide and it is still under consideration for global public health. There are many causes of conjunctivitis and difference clinical managements have to be provided for different causes. The interesting group of conjunctivitis disorders is those found in tropical zone. There are many tropical infections and disorders that can induce conjunctivitis and those problems are called tropical conjunctivitis. The problem can be infectious or non-infectious disorder. In this short article, the authors will summarize and discuss on important kinds of tropical conjunctivitis focusing on diagnosis and management.

IMPORTANT TROPICAL CONJUNCTIVITIS

1. *Tropical endemic limbo-conjunctivitis*
   Tropical endemic limbo-conjunctivitis is an important kind of conjunctivitis. Sometimes, it is called vernal conjunctivitis. Tropical endemic limboconjunctivitis can be considered an allergic conjunctivitis [2]. It usually affects males more frequently than females and the problem is common in warm and dry environments [2]. Chenge et al. noted that "the disease was equally distributed among sexes and the palpebral form was the most frequently encountered [3]" and "complications are uncommon [3]." According to the report on a large case series by et al., "allergy and past family history of tropical endemic limbo conjunctivitis are rare and filariasis is an aggravating factor of the disease [4]." Banla et al. noted that "allergy testing is of great importance for patients with frequent acute exacerbations" of tropical endemic limbo-conjunctivitis [5].
2. *Malarial conjunctivitis*
   Malaria is an important tropical infection that is caused by parasite, *Plasmodium spp*. The mosquito bite is the main mode of transmission. Malaria can cause several clinical presentations. Conjunctivitis can also be seen in malaria but it is usually seen as an adverse effect of antimarial drug use [6].
3. *Chikungunya conjunctivitis*
   Chikungunya infection is another important tropical infection that is caused by Chikungunya virus. Similar to malaria, the mosquito bite is the main mode of transmission. Chikungunya infection can cause several clinical presentations. Conjunctivitis is an important manifestation of Chikungunya infection. Fever, headache, arthralgia, myalgia and conjunctivitis are common [7]. Ng et al. noted that four-tenths of the patients with Chikungunya infections have conjunctivitis [8]. There is no specific treatment for Chikungunya infection as well as its ocular manifestation, conjunctivitis. However, as a viral infection, the self - limitation and spontaneous recovery is possible.

4. *Dengue conjunctivitis*
   Dengue infection is another important tropical infection that is caused by dengue virus. Similar to malaria and Chikungunya, the mosquito bite is the main mode of transmission. Dengue infection can cause several clinical presentations. Apart from acute febrile illness with hemorrhage, conjunctivitis is another important manifestation of dengue infection. Nearly 63 % of the patients have conjunctivitis [9]. According to the report on clinical manifestation of dengue by Buchy et al., "the most common presenting symptom was headache, followed by conjunctivitis, petechial rash, muscle and joint pain, nausea and abdominal pain [10]." There is no specific treatment for dengue infection as well as its ocular manifestation, conjunctivitis. However, as a viral infection, the self - limitation and spontaneous recovery is possible. For the severe case, the intense fluid replacement therapy is needed.
5. *Zika conjunctivitis*
   Zika infection is another important tropical infection that is caused by a flavirus. This infection is a new infection firstly identified in tropical Micronesia. Zika infection can induce mild disease characterized by rash, arthralgia, and conjunctivitis [11 - 12].
6. *Trachoma*
   Trachoma is an important tropical ocular infection caused by *Chlamydia trachomatis* [13 – 14]. Repeated inflammation can be seen and can result in scarring with can lead to blindness [13 – 14]. Castan et al. noted that 4 % of all tropical conjunctivitis was due to *C. trachomatis infection* [15]. For treatment, "intracellular acting agents such as doxycycline, macrolides like azithromycin and erythromycin and certain quinolones (i.e. levofloxacin and ofloxacin)" are the drug of choice [13].

CONCLUSION

There are many disorders in the group of tropical conjunctivitis. Due to the rapid globalization, the tropical conjunctivitis can be seen in the area outside the tropical zone. It is suggested that all practitioners should consider tropical conjunctivitis when they have to deal with any cases presenting with conjunctivitis.

REFERENCES

[1] Kappagoda, S; Ioannidis, JP. Neglected tropical diseases, survey and geometry of randomised evidence. *BMJ.*, 2012 Oct 22, 345, e6512.

[2] Koki, G; Omgbwa, Eballe, A; Epee, E; Njuenwet, Njapdunke, SB; Souleymanou, Wadjiri, Y; Bella, Assumpta, L; Ebana, Mvogo, C. Tropical endemic limboconjunctivitis (vernal conjunctivitis) in northern Cameroon. *J Fr Ophtalmol.*, 2011 Feb, 34(2), 113-7.

[3] Chenge, B; Makumyamviri, AM; Kaimbo, WA; Kaimbo, D. Tropical endemic limbo-conjunctivitis in Lúbumbashi, Democratic Republic of the Congo. *Bull Soc Belge Ophtalmol.*, 2003, (290), 9-16.

[4] Moukouri, dit, Nyolo, E; Nyolo, D; McMoli, T; Ndombo, K. Tropical endemic limbal conjunctivitis in Cameroon patients. Apropos of 819 cases in Yaounde. *Bull Soc Pathol Exot.*, 1993, 86(2), 120-4.

[5] Banla, M; Maneh, N; Vonor, B; Nonon, Saa, KB; Agba, A; Gantin, RG; Balo, KP; Soboslay, PT; Bakondé, B. Tropical endemic limbo-conjunctivitis (TELC) and allergic management, a preliminary study in Togolese children. *J Fr Ophtalmol.*, 2013 Oct, 36(8), 677-82.

[6] Moussala, M; Binam, F; Nkam, M; Kouda, Zeh, A; Bengono, G. Ocular manifestations and sequelae of Lyell syndrome caused by sulfadoxine-pyrimethamine in Cameroon. *Ophtalmol.*, 1998 Jan, 21(1), 72-7.

[7] Ahrenstorf, G; Burkhardt, O; Witte, T; Stoll, M; Schmidt, RE. Chikungunya, fever and joint pains after vacation in a tropical area. *Dtsch Med Wochenschr.*, 2008 Feb, 133(9), 406-8.

[8] Ng, LF; Chow, A; Sun, YJ; Kwek, DJ; Lim, PL; Dimatatac, F; Ng, LC; Ooi, EE; Choo, KH; Her, Z; Kourilsky, P; Leo, YS. IL-1beta, IL-6, and RANTES as biomarkers of Chikungunya severity. *PLoS One.*, 2009, 4(1), e4261.

[9] Harn, MR. Clinical study on dengue fever during 1987-1988 epidemic at Kaohsiung City, southern Taiwan. *Gaoxiong Yi Xue Ke Xue Za Zhi.*, 1989 Jan, 5(1), 58-65.

[10] Buchy, P; Vo, VL; Bui, KT; Trinh, TX; Glaziou, P; Le, TT; Le, VL; Bui, TC. Secondary dengue virus type 4 infections in Vietnam. *Southeast Asian J Trop Med Public Health.*, 2005 Jan, 36(1), 178-85.

[11] Hayes, EB. Zika virus outside Africa. *Emerg Infect Dis.*, 2009 Sep, 15(9), 1347-50.

[12] Duffy, MR; Chen, TH; Hancock, WT; Powers, AM; Kool, JL; Lanciotti, RS; Pretrick, M; Marfel, M; Holzbauer, S; Dubray, C; Guillaumot, L; Griggs, A; Bel, M; Lambert, AJ; Laven, J; Kosoy, O; Panella, A;

Biggerstaff, BJ, Fischer, M; Hayes, EB. Zika virus outbreak on Yap Island, Federated States of Micronesia. *N Engl J Med.*, 2009 Jun 11, 360(24), 2536-43.

[13] Stock, I; Henrichfreise, B. Infections with Chlamydia trachomatis. *Med Monatsschr Pharm.*, 2012 Jun, 35(6), 209-22.

[14] Burton, MJ. Trachoma, an overview. *Br Med Bull.*, 2007, 84, 99-116.

[15] Castan, R; Resnikoff, S; Guillemot, de, Liniers, F; Huguet, P; Peyramaure, F. Tropical conjunctivitis, infectious etiology and validation of its clinical features. *Rev Int Trach Pathol Ocul Trop Subtrop Sante Publique.*, 1991, 68, 63-73.

INDEX

A

D

H

I

J

K

L

M

N

O

P

Q

R

S

T

U

V

W

X

Y

Z